I0768185

The stability ball is a must have piece of equipment for an at home gym. They go by many other names: fitness ball, yoga ball, exercise ball, Swiss ball and physio ball. For the purpose of this book, I will use the term 'stability ball' as I believe one of the main benefits is that they help train your stabilizer muscles and improve balance. They're both affordable and portable as they are just made of a lightweight vinyl and can be easily filled with air with a small pump. Although stability balls can be used in conjunction with other equipment, this book features 100 exercises using only the stability ball to achieve a total body workout for all ability levels. Be mindful of the notations regarding difficulty and required skills as it most certainly possible to get injured on a stability ball. They do roll and require balance…you can fall off. It's a good idea to use caution as you get used to the various movements by positioning yourself on top of an exercise mat or near a wall to help with footing or a stable surface to hold onto. Also important that you have enough space to use it safely. Ie; you don't want to fall and crash into a table or lamp. It's also important that you find the right size. They do come in a range of options.

Height 4'8"-5'3" > Ball Size 55cm
Height 5'4"-5'10" > Ball Size 65cm
Height 5'11"-6'4" > Ball Size 75cm

Keep in mind that a smaller ball is a larger challenge. So it is ok to use a larger or smaller ball than indicated by this chart depending on your fitness level. This book is intended only for those who have received medical clearance to do so. Please be aware that any exercise or physical activity program comes with a possibility of physical injury and choosing to engage in this exercise program is done so at your own risk.

<u>1. Half Moon</u>
Beginner

From a kneeling position, seat the butt back onto the heels. Hold the stability ball in both hands and raise the arms straight up overhead. To perform this exercise, you will lean over to one side, allowing the stability ball to lead. Then raise back up to the start position and repeat on the other side. This completes one rep.

What it Works: While the arms and shoulders will be engaged as they hold the stability ball above the head, this exercise primarily focuses on the side abdominal muscles (or obliques.)

Begin with 1 set of 10 reps, building to 3 sets of 10 reps.

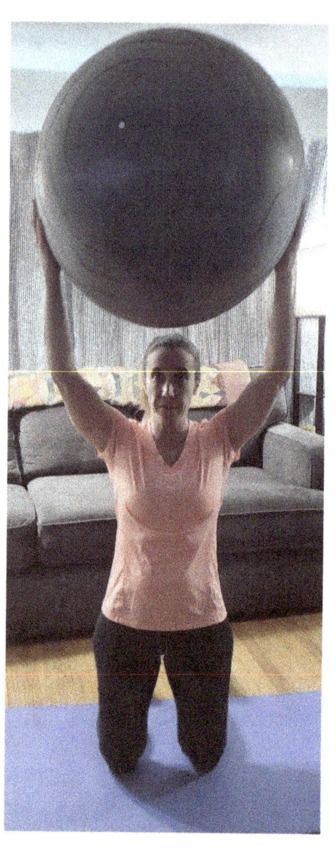 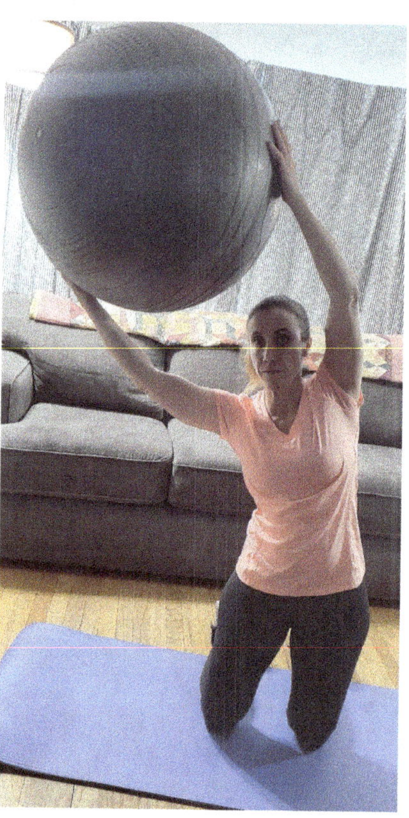

<u>2. Wipers</u>
Beginner

Lie down on your back on the floor with the stability ball positioned between the feet. Extend the legs up straight. Reach your arms out to either side with palms down to help support the body through this movement. To perform this exercise, you will lower the legs over to one side by twisting at the waist but being careful to keep the hips on the floor. Engage the obliques to pull the legs back up to center, then repeat on the other side. This completes one rep.

What it Works: This exercise primarily targets the lower (or transverse) abs and the obliques.

Begin with 1 set of 10 reps, building to 3 sets of 10 reps.

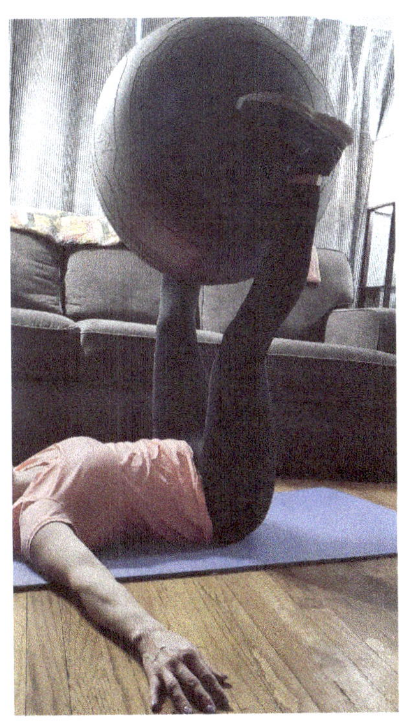
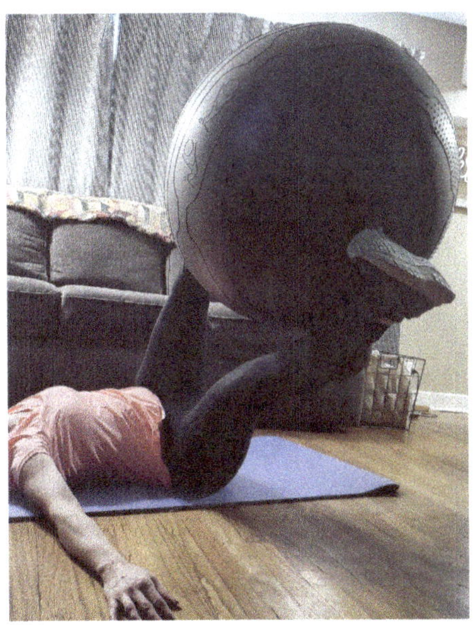

<u>3. Supine Leg Twists</u>
Beginner

Lie on your back on the floor with the stability ball between both feet. The back and hands will be anchored to the floor throughout. Extend the straight legs up between a 45 and 90 degree angle. To perform this exercise, you will twist the legs to one side while keeping the lower back anchored to the floor. Return to center and repeat on the other side. This completes one rep.

What it Works: This exercise focuses on the lower (or transverse) abs and the obliques.

Begin with 1 set of 10 reps, building to 3 sets of 10 reps.

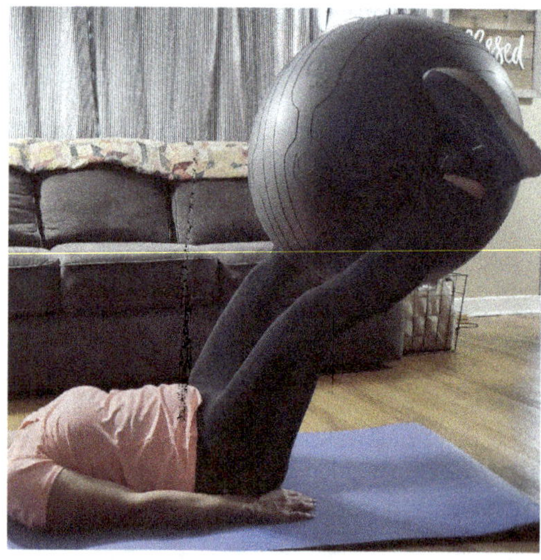

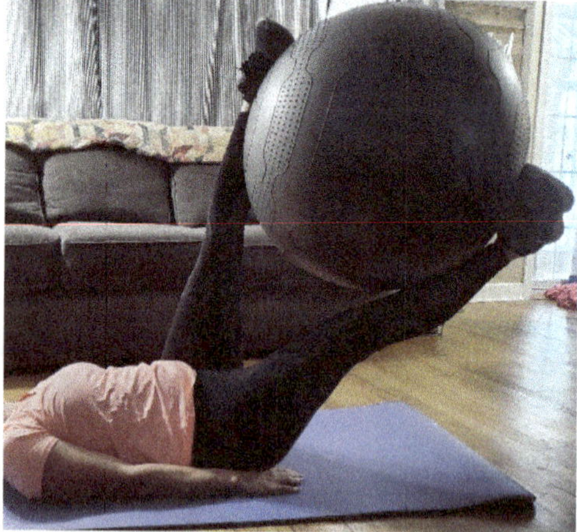

<u>4. Lateral Pelvic Tilts</u>
Beginner

Sit on the stability ball with the knees bent, feet flat on the floor, back straight and hands on the hips. To perform this exercise, roll the ball out to one side by tilting the pelvis over to the side while keeping the upper body up straight. Return to the center and repeat to the other side. This is one rep.

What it Works: This exercise mainly focuses on the stabilizer muscles of the hips as well as the muscles of the lower back and lower abdominals.

Begin with 1 reps.   set of 10 reps, building to up to 4 sets of 15

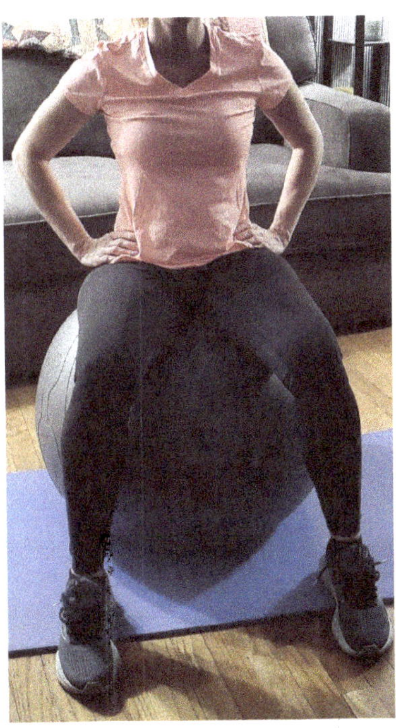
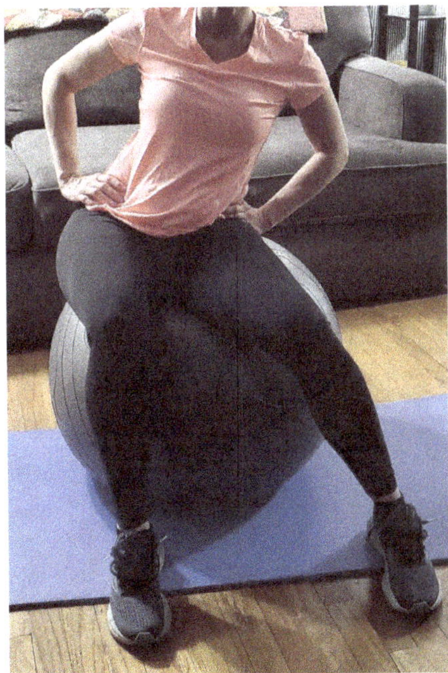

<u>5. Seated Toe Taps</u>
Beginner

From a seated position, you will have the legs out straight and you will hold the stability ball in both hands with arms stretched out straight. The ball will be at eye level throughout. To perform this exercise you will raise one leg up straight so that the top of the foot touches the bottom of the stability ball. Lower back down and repeat on the other side. This completes one rep.

What it Works: This exercise focuses on the lower abdominal muscles as well as the muscles at the top, front of the leg (or hip flexors.)

Begin with 1 set of 10 reps, building to 3 sets of 10 reps.

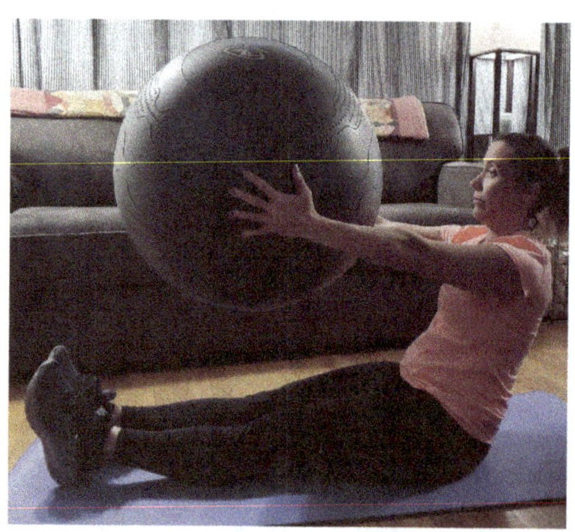
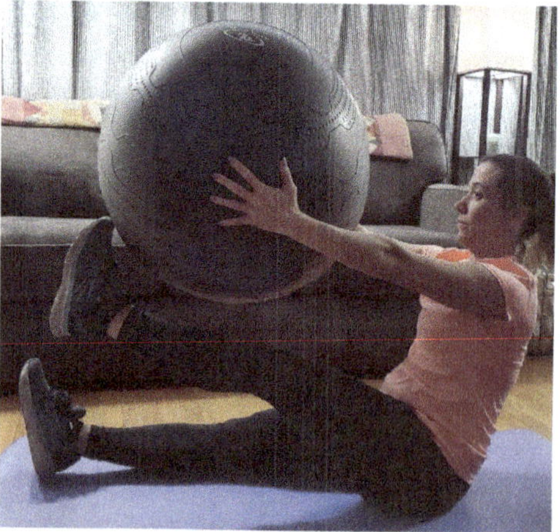

<u>6. Seated Leg Balance</u>
Beginner - Intermediate

You will be seated on the stability ball with the body up straight and the knees bent at a 90 degree angle. The fingertips will be at the temples with the elbows extended out wide (or a beginner modification would be to keep the hands on the stability ball.) To perform this exercise, you will straighten one leg up while keeping the other foot anchored to the floor. Hold this position for 5 seconds while trying to keep the body as still as possible before lowering back down. Repeat on the other side. This makes one rep.

What it Works: Although the hip flexors do need to work to raise the leg, this is a lower core exercise. The transverse abs, hips and lower back are the primary focus.

Begin with 1 set of 5 reps, building to 3 sets of 10 reps.

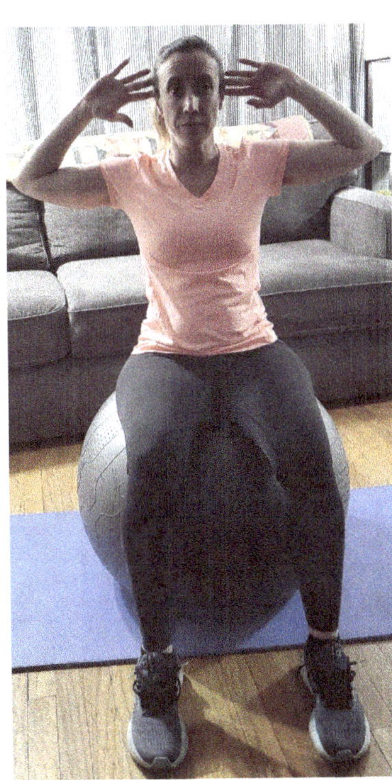 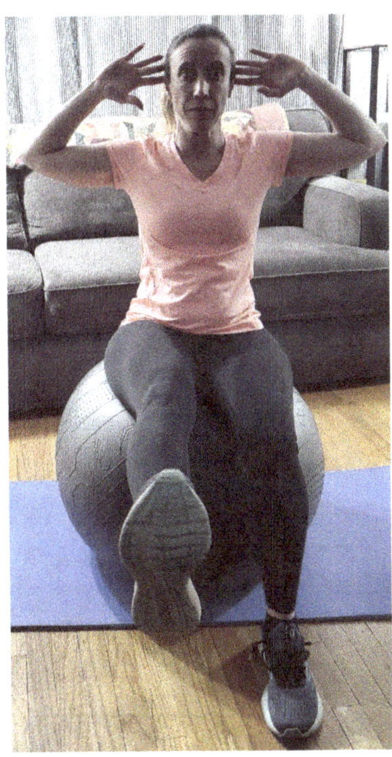

<u>7. Dead Bug</u>
Beginner - Intermediate

Lie on your back with knees bent at 90 degrees and arms stretched up straight towards the ceiling. The stability ball will be in the center, supported by the knees and arms. This is the starting position. To perform this exercise, you will extend one leg out straight so that it hovers above the floor while simultaneously lowering the opposite arm down above the head to hover above the floor. The opposing arm and leg will be supporting the stability ball. Return to the start position and repeat on the opposite side. This is one rep.

What it Works: This is an abominal exercise that specifically targets the rectus abdominis and engages the obliques as well.

Begin with 1 set of 5 reps, building up to 3 sets of 15 reps.

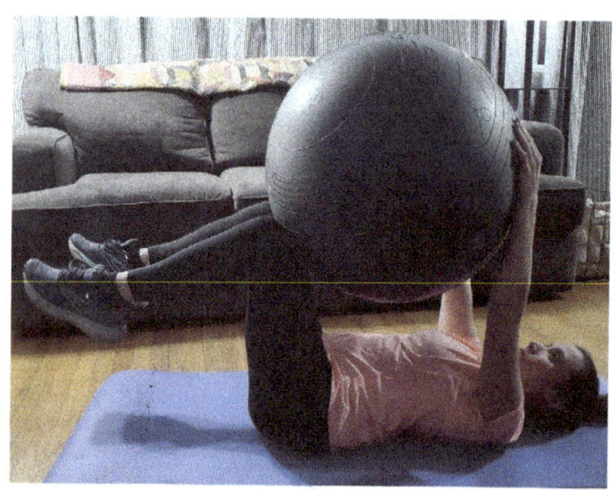

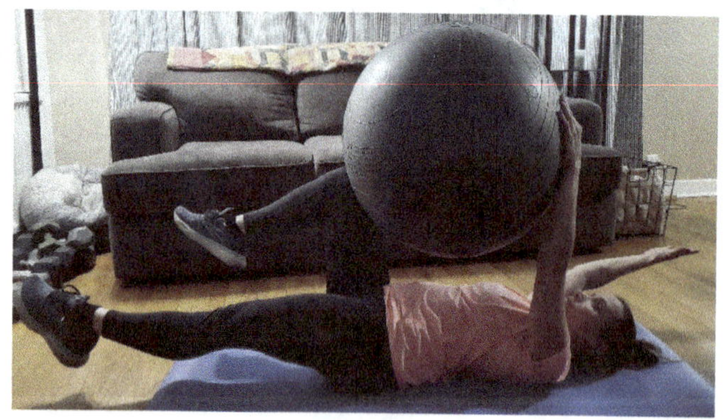

<u>8. Ball Squeeze Leg Lifts</u>
Beginner - Intermediate

Lying on your back on the floor, place the stability ball between both feet and squeeze.   You are going to put your arms very close to the body to help stabilize. To perform this exercise, raise the legs slightly so the ball hovers above the ground. Raise the legs to a maximum 90 degree angle before lowering back down to hover. This completes one rep.

What it Works: This is mainly an abdominal exercise that concentrates on the lower abs, but the hip flexors (on the upper part of the front of the legs) are heavily engaged as well.

Begin with 1 seat of 10 reps, building to 3 sets of 10 reps.

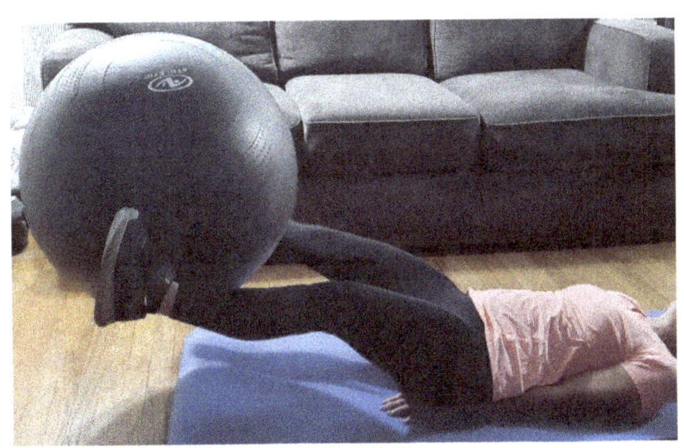

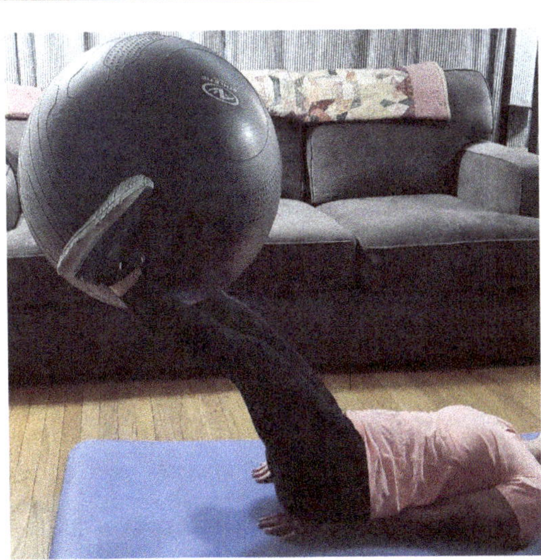

<u>9. Crunch with Legs on Stability Ball</u>
Beginner

Lay flat on your back with your knees bent at 90 degrees and the calves resting on the stability ball. With your finger tips at the temples and elbows bent out wide, you are going to raise the chest off the floor and in towards the knees. Be careful not to pull on the head or neck. This is not a huge range of motion. You are crunching in until you feel the abdominal muscles contract, then lowering back down to the start position. This is one rep.

What it Works: This is an abdominal exercise. It specifically targets the muscles of the rectus abdominis.

Begin with 1 set of 10 reps, building to up to 4 sets of 15 reps.

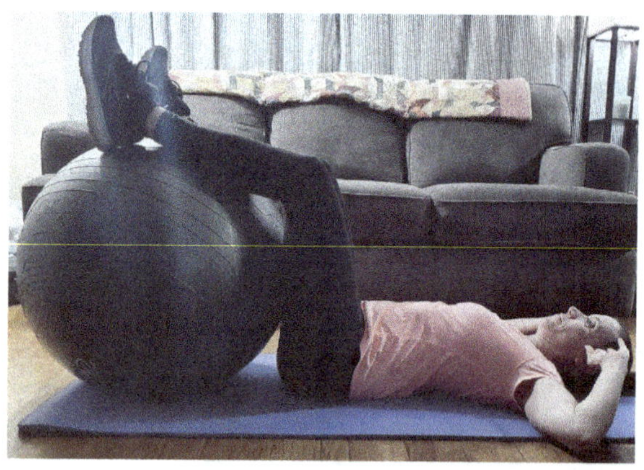

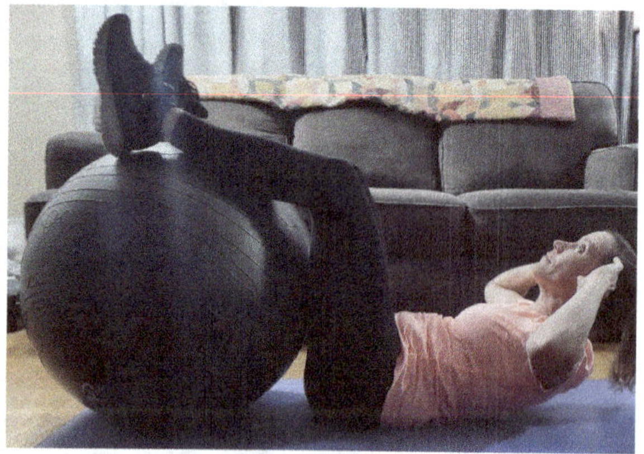

<u>10. Reverse Crunch</u>
Beginner

Lie flat on your back with your knees bent at 90 degrees and resting on top of the stability ball. The arms will be lying flat against the sides of the body throughout. Separate the legs so the stability ball can be squeezed between them. To perform this exercise, you will contract your abs and curl your hips and knees in towards your chest while pushing down through your palms. Roll back down to the start position. This completes one rep.

What it Works: This is an abdominal exercise that specifically targets the transverse abdominals.

Begin with 1 set of 10 reps, building to 4 sets of 10 reps.

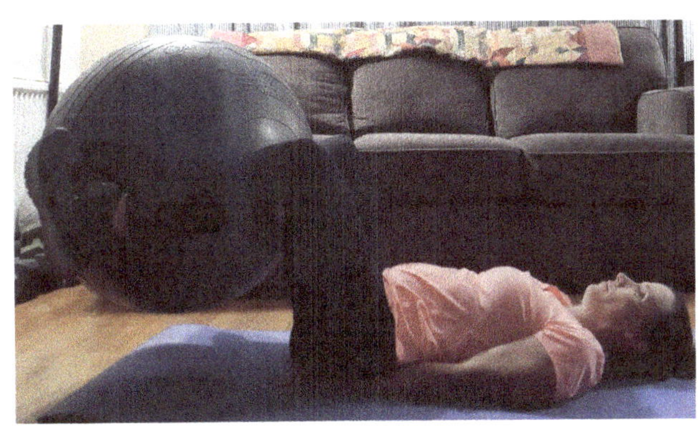

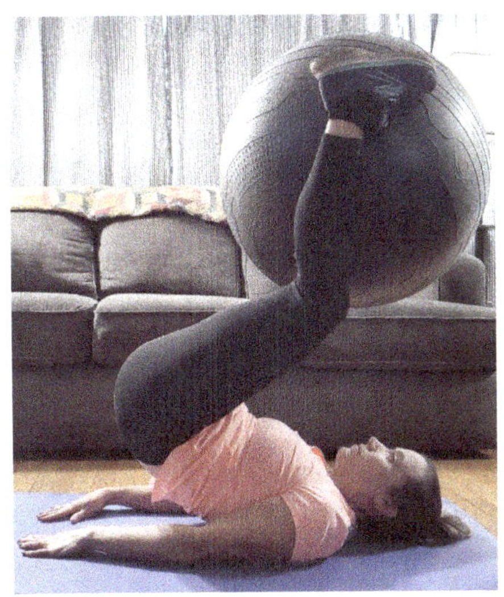

<u>11. Long Arm Oblique Twist</u>
Beginner

Lay flat on your back with your knees bent at 90 degrees and the calves resting on the stability ball. Extend the arms straight up in front of the chest and clasp the hands together. To perform this exercise, you will crunch in while bringing the hands over to the side of the opposite knees. Roll back down to the start position and repeat on the other side. This completes one rep.

What it Works: This is an abdominal exercise. It specifically targets the rectus abdominis and the obliques.

Begin with 1 set of 5 reps, building to 3 sets of 10 reps.

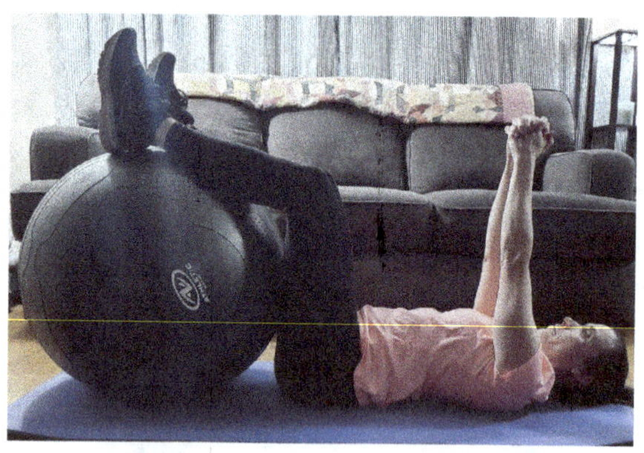

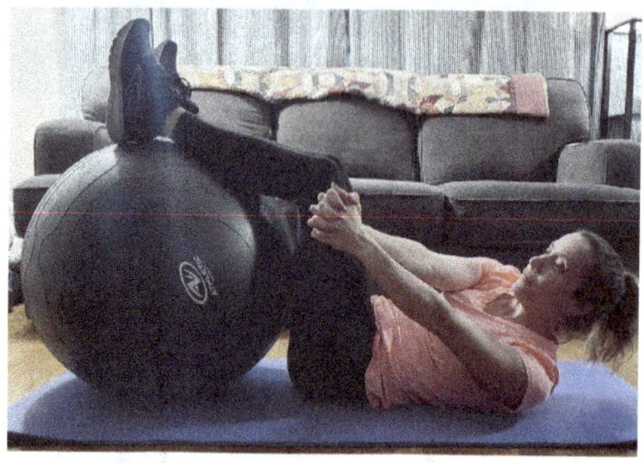

<u>12. Overhead Rotation Crunch</u>
Beginner

Lie on your back with knees bent and feet flat on the floor. Hold the stability ball in both hands and extend the arms overhead. To perform this exercise you will crunch the abs in while reaching the arms across the body bringing the stability ball to the opposite side next to the knees. Roll the body back down to the start position and repeat on the opposite side. This completes one rep.

What it Works: This is an abdominal exercise that focuses on the rectus abdominis and the obliques.

Begin with 1 set of 5 reps, building to 3 sets of 10 reps.

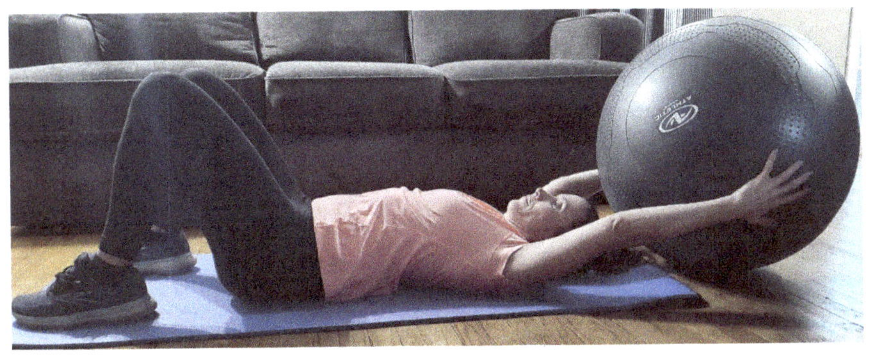

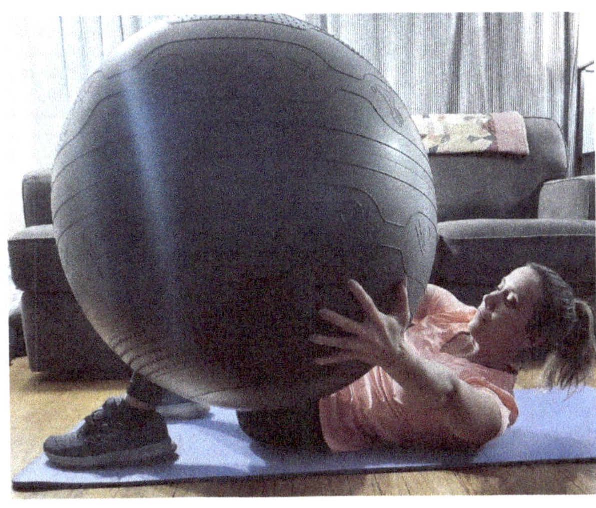

<u>13. Ball Walk Outs</u>
Beginner

Sit on the stability ball with the knees bent at 90 degrees, body up straight and the fingers at the temples with the elbows out wide. (As a beginner, the hands can press against the stability ball instead.) To perform this exercise, walk the feet forward while rolling the ball up the back. Stop when the ball has reached the head and shoulders and the body is in a flat table top position. Walk back to the start position. This completes one rep.

What it Works: This is an abdominal exercise that targets the rectus abdominis and transverse abs.

Begin with 1 set of 5 reps, building to 3 sets of 15 reps.

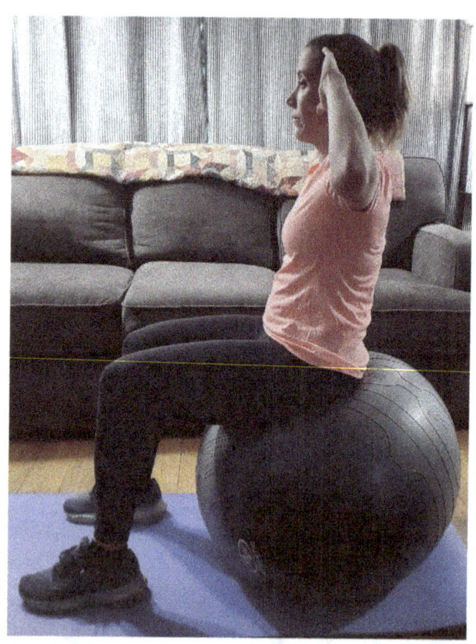

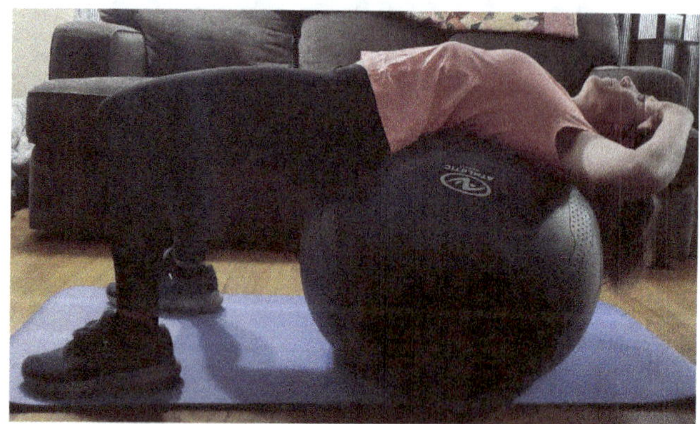

<u>14. Knee Raise</u>
Intermediate

From a seated position on the stability ball, roll the ball out so the feet are flat on the floor, knees are bent at 90 degrees, torso is parallel with the floor and the stability ball is under the back and hips. Fingertips will be at temples with elbows out wide. This is the starting position. To perform this exercise, you will raise one knee straight up. Do not allow the hips to move out to the sides. Lower back down and repeat with the other leg. This is one rep.

What it Works: This exercise primarily targets the lower or transverse abs.

Begin with 1 set of 10 reps, building up to 4 sets of 15 reps

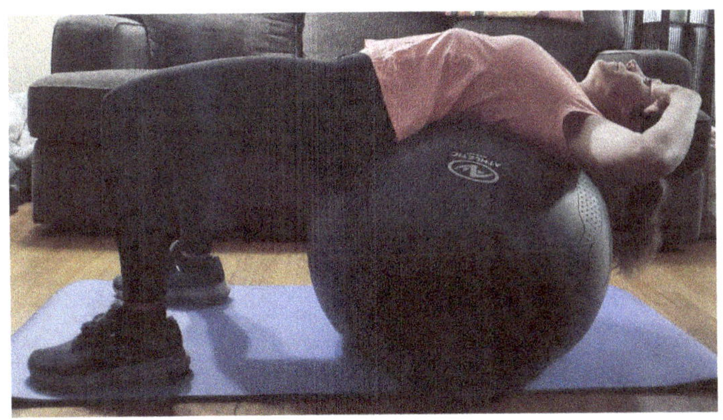

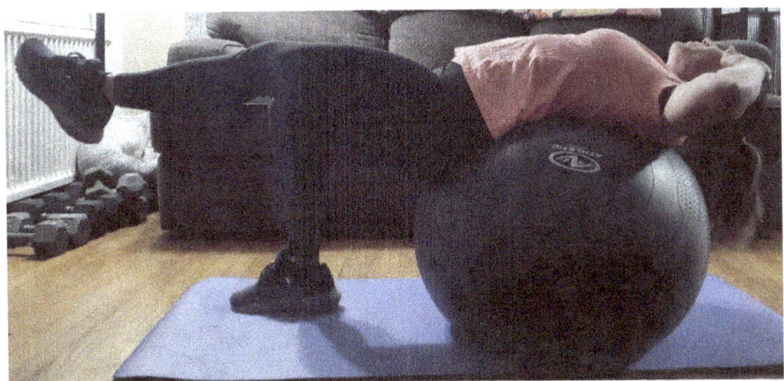

<u>15. Alternating Crossovers</u>
Intermediate

From a seated position on the stability ball, roll the ball out so the feet are flat on the floor, knees are bent at 90 degrees, torso is parallel with the floor and the stability ball is under the back and hips. The arms will be angled back and to the sides helping to stabilize the body. To perform this exercise, you will extend one leg straight up while simultaneously reaching the opposite arm straight up towards the foot of the extended leg. Lower back to the start position and repeat on the other side. This completes one rep.

What it Works: This exercise mainly focuses on the abdominals (transverse, rectus abdominis and obliques) but the shoulders, chest and hip flexors are engaged as well.

Begin with 1 set of 5 reps, building to 3 sets of 10 reps.

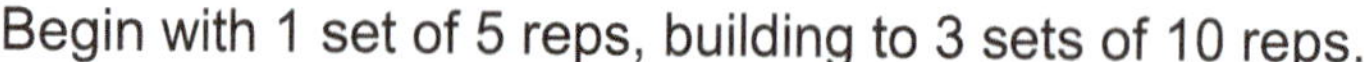

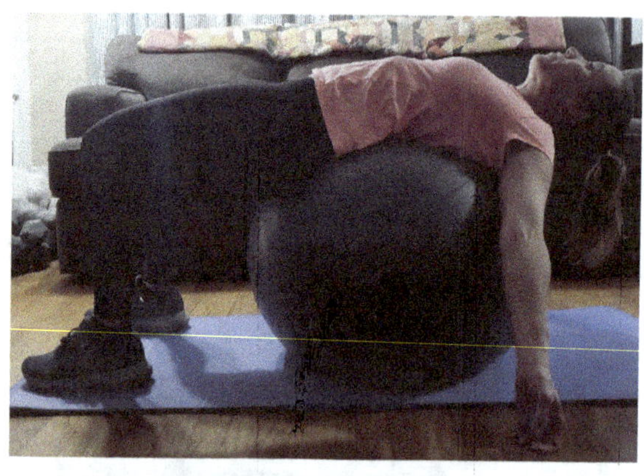

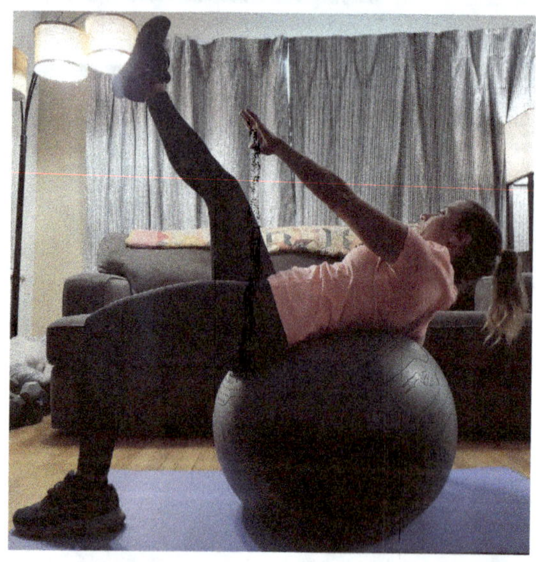

<u>16. Supine Single Knee-Ins with a Twist</u>
Beginner

Lie flat on your back with legs extended out straight and the stability ball in both hands extended up above the chest. Curling the torso up, reach the ball forward while lifting one leg off the ground and bending it in while simultaneously twisting the torso towards that knee and extending the ball out to the side of it. The bottom leg should remain anchored to the floor throughout. Lower back to the start position. This completes one rep. Repeat evenly on each side.

What it Works: The hip flexors (the upper part of the front of the leg) are working during this exercise, but it is primarily an abdominal exercise (transverse, rectus abdominis and obliques.)

Begin with 1 set of 5 reps, building to 3 sets of 10 reps.

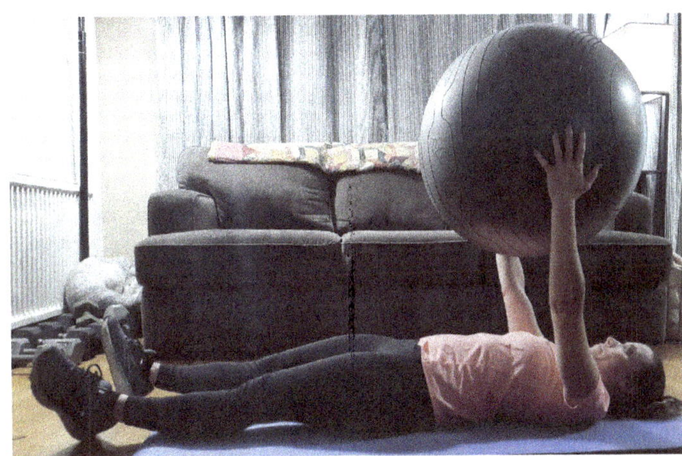

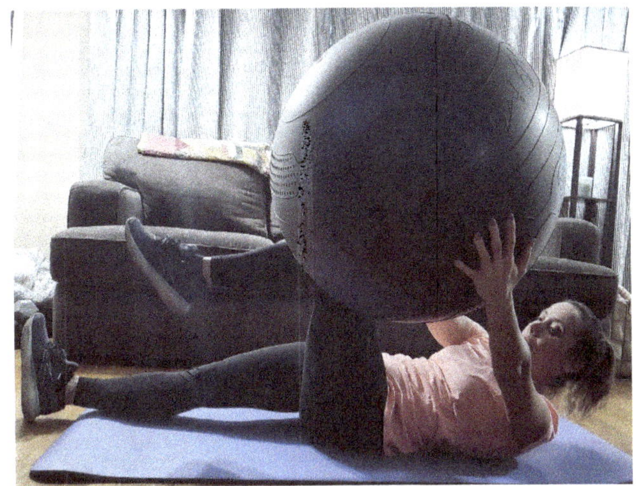

<u>17. Abdominal Crunch</u>
Beginner

From a seated position on the stability ball, roll the ball out so the feet are flat on the floor, knees are bent at 90 degrees, torso is parallel with the floor and the stability ball is under the back and hips. Fingertips will be at temples with elbows out wide. You will curl the torso up by contracting the abdominal muscles and driving the heels down into the floor. This does not need to be a big range of motion and be careful not to pull the neck or stretch the chin forward. Return down to the start position. This is one rep.

What it Works: This exercise concentrates on the abdominal muscles. Specifically the rectus abdominis.

Begin with 1 set of 5 reps, building to 3 sets of 5 reps, then eventually up to 4 sets of 15 reps.

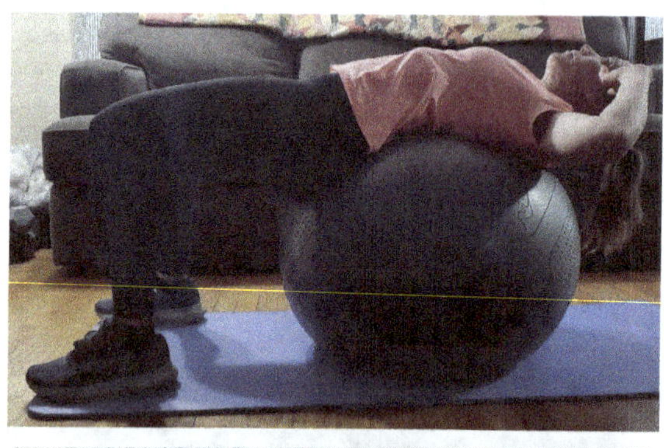

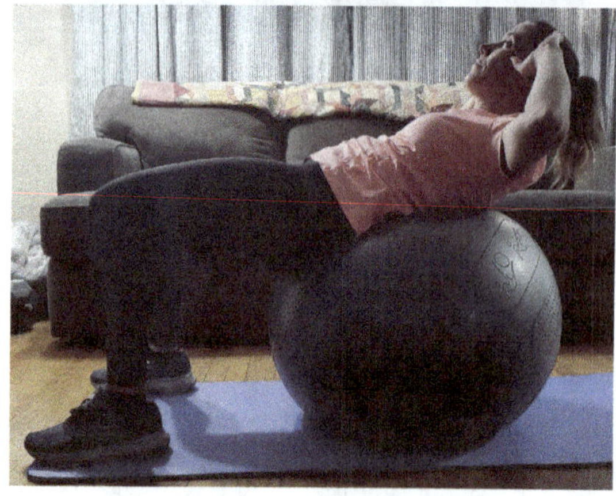

<u>18. Crunch with Leg Lift</u>
Intermediate

From a seated position on the stability ball, roll the ball out so the feet are flat on the floor, knees are bent at 90 degrees, torso is parallel with the floor and the stability ball is under the back and hips. Fingertips will be at temples with elbows out wide. You will curl the torso up by contracting the abdominal muscles and driving one heel down into the floor as the opposite knee marches in towards the torso. Lower back down and complete with the other leg. This completes one rep.

What it Works: This exercise concentrates on the abdominis rectus and the transverse abs.

Begin with 1 set of 5 reps, building to 3 sets of 10 reps.

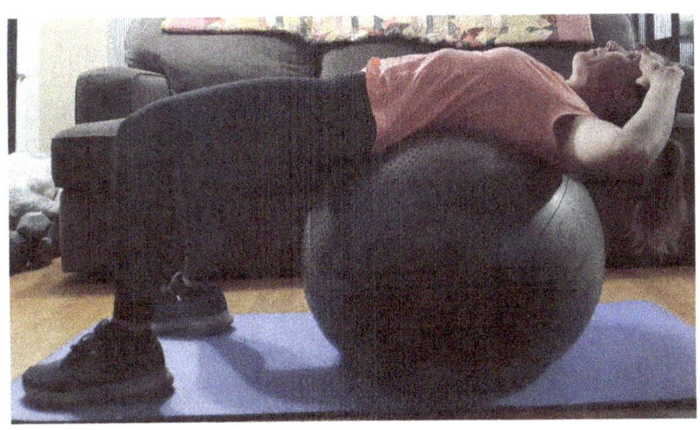

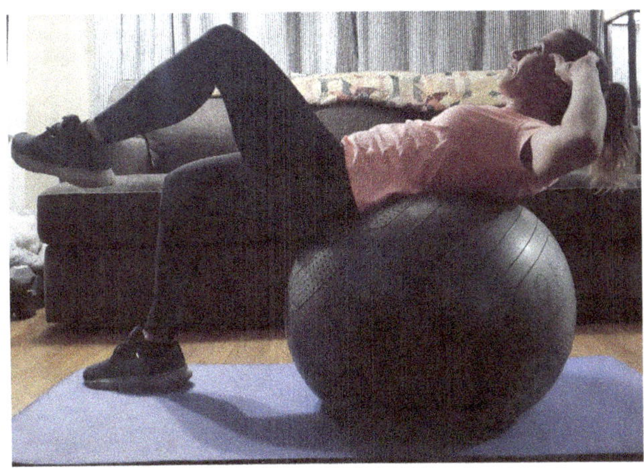

<u>19. Crunch Twists</u>
Beginner

From a seated position on the stability ball, roll the ball out so the feet are flat on the floor, knees are bent at 90 degrees, torso is parallel with the floor and the stability ball is under the back and hips. Fingertips will be at temples with elbows out wide. You will curl the torso up by contracting the abdominal muscles and driving the heels down into the floor. As you crunch up, you will twist your body over to one side, leading with the shoulder. Lower back down to the start position and repeat on the other side. This is one rep.

What it Works: This exercise concentrates on the abdominal muscles (the rectus abdominis, transverse abdominis and obliques.)

Begin with 1 set of 5 reps, building to 3 sets of 5 reps, then eventually up to 4 sets of 15 reps.

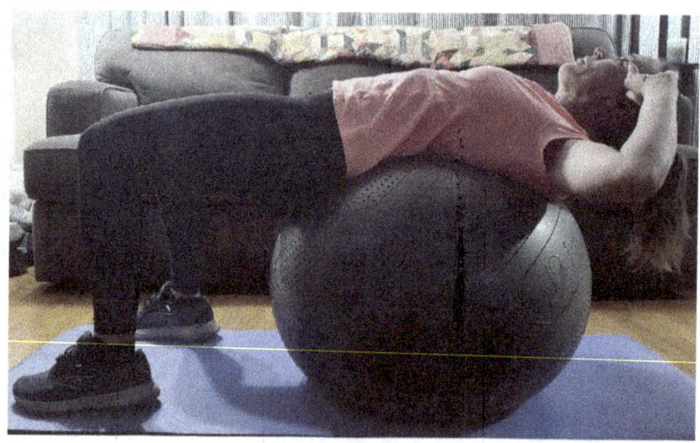

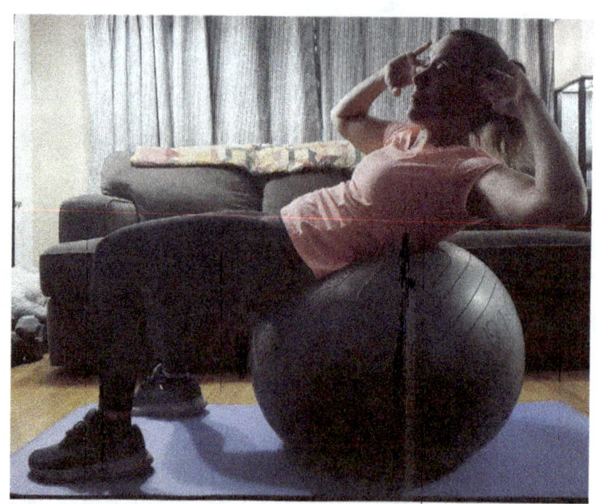

<u>20. Long Arm Crunch</u>
Intermediate

From a seated position on the stability ball, roll the ball out so the feet are flat on the floor, knees are bent at 90 degrees, torso is parallel with the floor and the stability ball is under the back and hips. Arms are extended overhead and clasped together. To perform this exercise you will keep the arms overhead throughout. Crunch the abs in while keeping the lower body still. Lower back to the start position. This is one rep.

What it Works: This is an abdominal exercise, targeting the rectus abdominis.

Begin with 1 set of 5 reps, building to 3 sets of 15 reps.

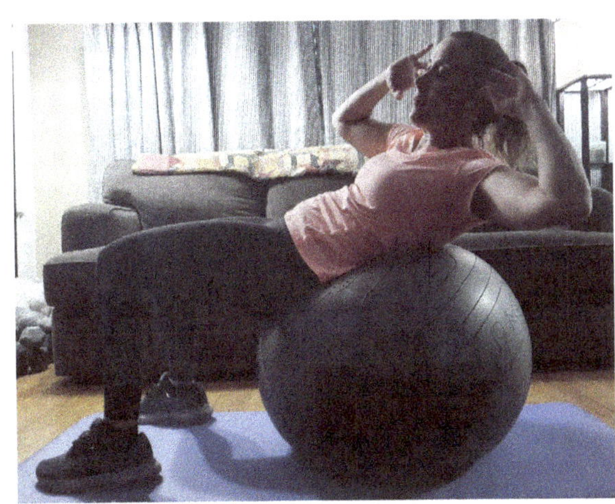

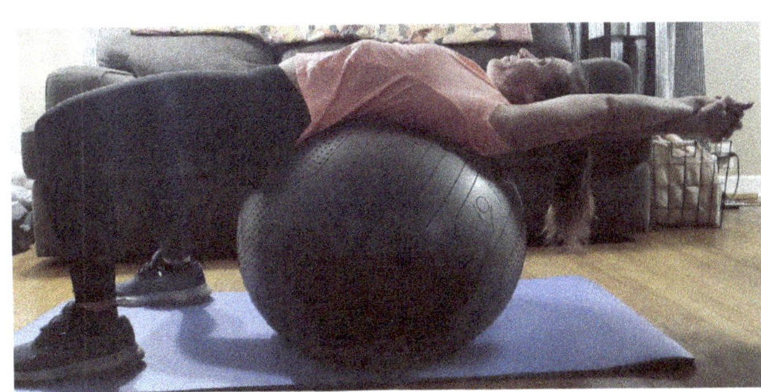

<u>21. Supine Long Arm Crunch</u>
Intermediate

Lie on your back so that your entire body is flat on the floor while holding the stability ball in both hands with the arms stretched out overhead. To perform this exercise, you will keep the lower body anchored to the floor throughout. The arms will stay stretched out while gripping the ball in both hands. You will roll the body up to a full sit up, keeping the arms stretched out above the head. Roll back down to the start position. This completes one rep.

What it Works: This is an abdominal exercise, targeting the rectus abdominis.

Begin with 1 set of 5 reps, building to 3 sets of 10 reps.

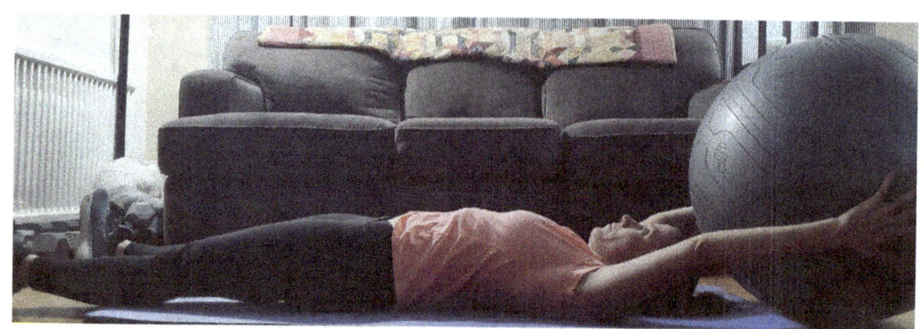

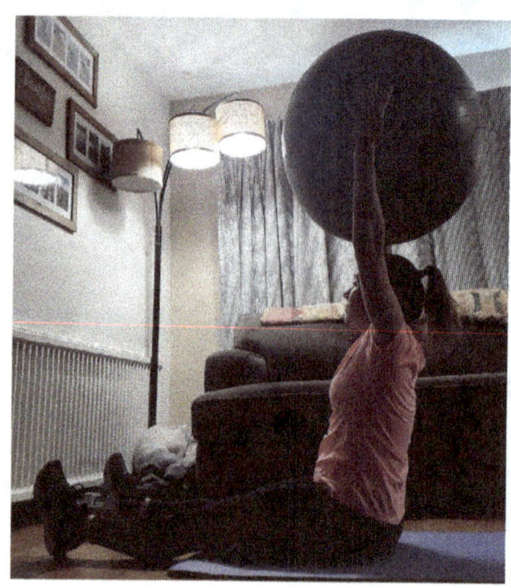

<u>22. Passover Crunch</u>
Intermediate

Lie on your back with the knees bent, feet flat on the floor and the stability ball between both hands with the arms stretched up straight overhead. Simultaneously bring the knees in towards the ball, meeting at the torso and transferring the stability ball from the hands to between the knees. Lower all the way back down before crunching back in and transferring the ball back to the hands. Lower back down to the start position. This is one rep.

What it Works: This exercise focuses on the abdominal muscles as well as the inner thigh or adductor muscles.

Begin with 1 set of 5 reps, building to 4 sets of 10 reps.

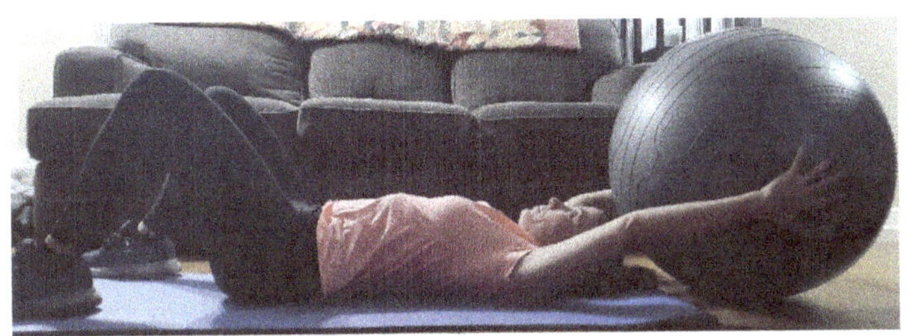

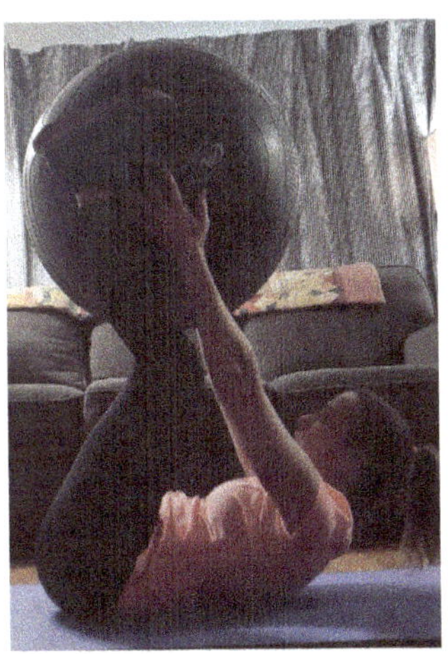

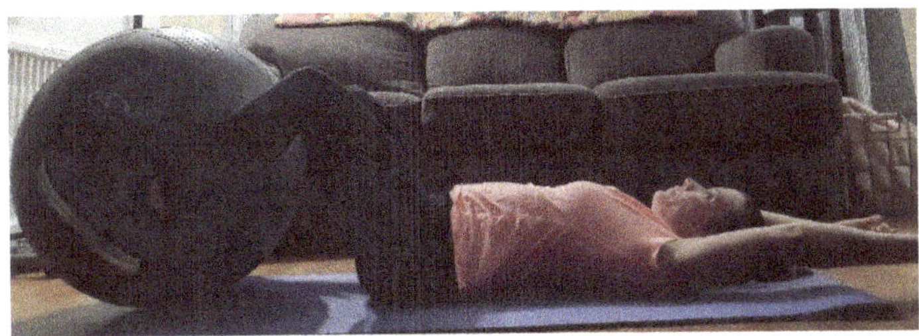

<u>23. Straight Leg Roll-Up</u>
Intermediate

Lie flat on your back on the floor with the heels resting on the stability ball and the arms stretched out straight in front of the chest. To perform this exercise, you will drive your heels down into the stability ball while rolling the body up and reaching your arms towards the toes. The goal is to touch the toes before rolling back down. This is one rep.

What it Works: This exercise targets the rectus abdominis.

Begin with 1 set of 5 reps, building to 4 sets of 10 reps.

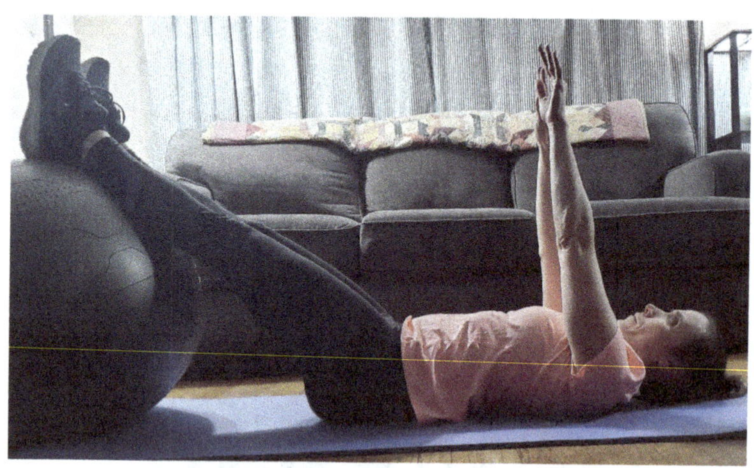

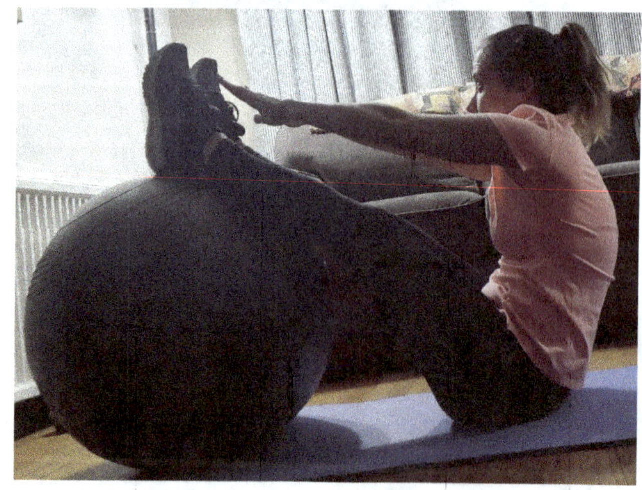

<u>24. Rope Climbers</u>
Intermediate

Position the stability ball so that it is under the hips and lower back and the knees are bent at 90 degrees with the feet flat on the floor. Lean the torso back to a 45 degree angle. To perform this exercise, you will reach the arms straight up and rotate them in such a way as to be climbing an imaginary rope. As one arm reaches up, the body should come to an upright position. Lower the torso back down and repeat on the other side. This completes one rep.

What it Works: This is an abdominal exercise that targets the rectus abdominis and obliques.

Begin with 1 set of 10 reps, building to 3 sets of 10 reps.

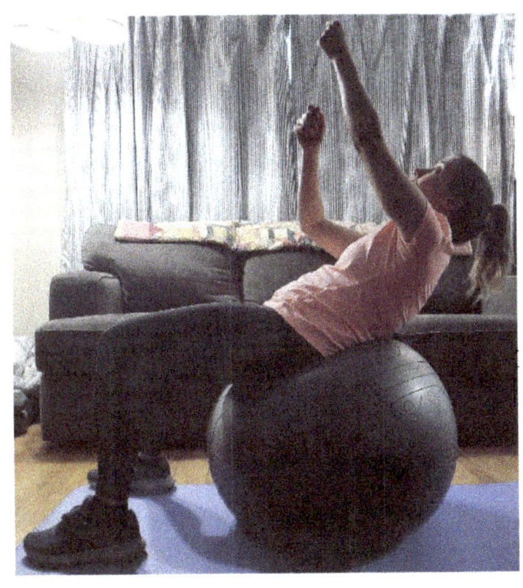

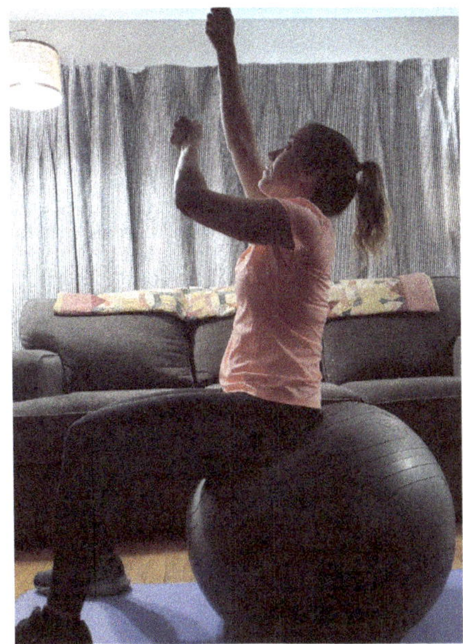

<u>25. Bicycles</u>
Beginner - Intermediate

Lie on your back with your fingertips at your temples and elbows bent out wlde. The stability ball will be positioned between the feet while the knees are bent and the legs are elevated off the floor. To perform this exercise, you will bring one knee in towards the chest while twisting the opposite shoulder in towards that knee. Lower back down to the start position and repeat on the other side. This is one rep.

What it Works: This exercise primarily works the abdominal muscles, including the rectus abdominis, the transverse abdominis and the obliques.

Begin with 1 set of 10 reps, building up to 3 sets of 15 reps.

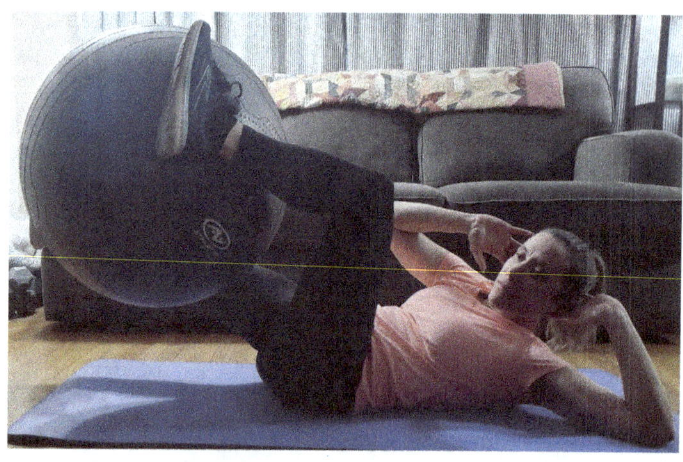

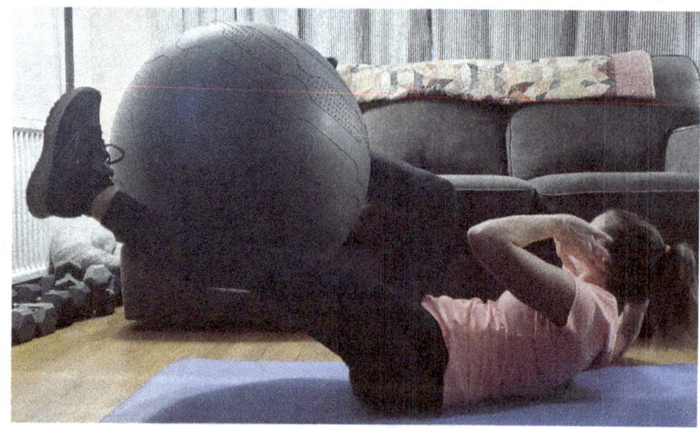

26. Lateral Crunch
Advanced

For this exercise, you will need to position yourself so that your feet are anchored against a wall and you are lying sideways with your hip resting on the stability ball. Your fingertips will be at the temples with elbows bent out to the side. To perform this exercise, you will raise your body up leading with the top elbow, pause then lower slowly back down to the start position. This completes one rep. Repeat evenly on each side.

What it Works: This exercise targets the obliques.

Begin with 1 set of 5 reps, building to 3 sets of 10 reps.

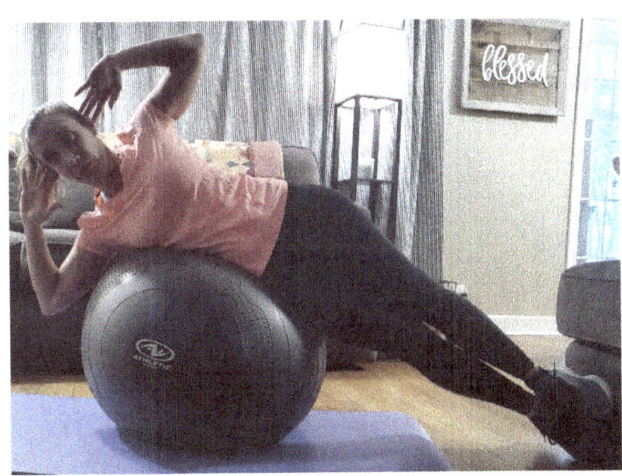

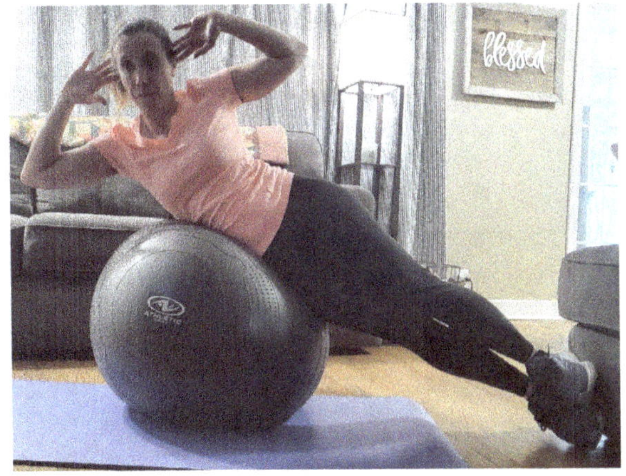

<u>27. Russian Twists</u>
Beginner

From a seated position, roll out so that the feet stay flat on the floor, knees are bent at 90 degrees and the back is resting on top of the stability ball. Press the palms together and extend the arms up straight above the chest. This is the starting position. The hips should stay stable and even throughout. To perform this exercise, you will rotate the torso over to one side by rolling onto the bottom shoulder as far as you can before returning to the start position. Repeat on the other side. This completes one rep.

What it Works: This core exercise especially targets the lower abs and the obliques.

Begin with 1 set of 5 reps, building up to 4 sets of 10 reps.

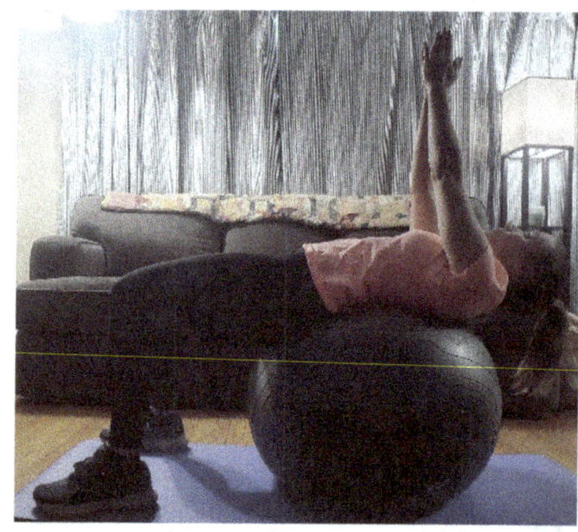

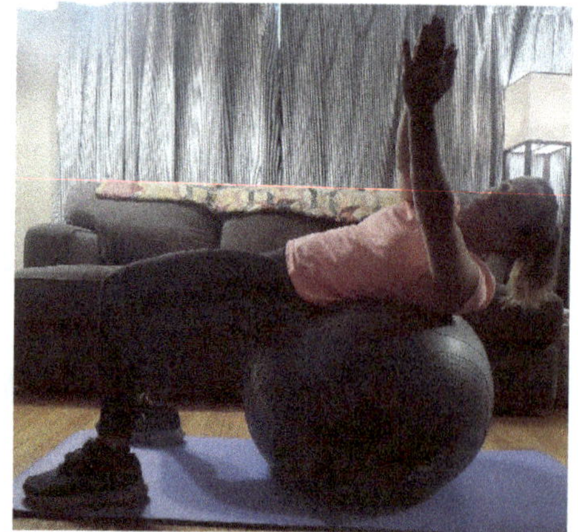

<u>28. Hover Plank</u>
Intermediate

This is a static exercise, meaning you will be holding one position. The forearms will be resting on the stability ball with the elbows under the shoulders. The body will be a straight line with the tailbone tucked, core braced and toes anchored to the floor. Hold this position without letting the stability ball roll or the back arch.

What it Works: This is a total body exercise as the glutes and shoulders must remain engaged throughout, but it is primarily an abdominal exercise as the rectus abdominis must work to maintain stability.

Begin by holding for 10 seconds for 1 rep, building up to 60 seconds for 3 reps.

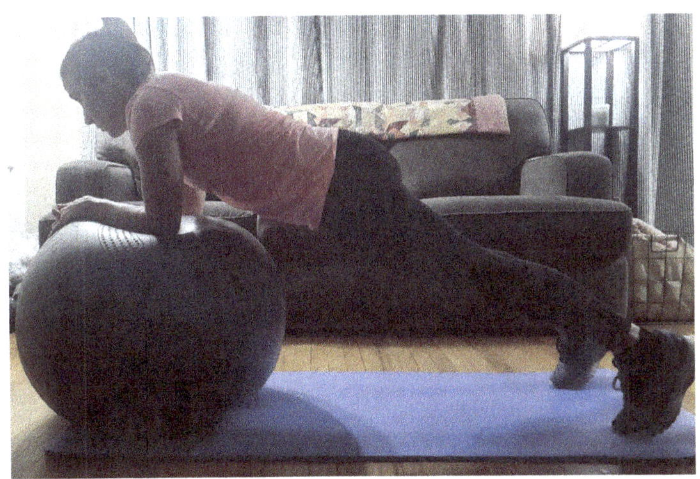

<u>29. Side Plank</u>
Intermediate-Advanced

This is a static exercise, meaning you will be holding one position. You will be on your side, with the bottom forearm and elbow resting on the stability ball. (This is an advanced move, so you have the option to drop the bottom knee to the floor as a modification). The body will be in a straight line from head to feet with the feet stacked on top of each other. Hold this position without letting the hips move up or down.

What it Works: This is a total body exercise, but it primarily works the obliques.

Begin by holding for 10 seconds for 1 rep, building up to 60 seconds for 3 reps.

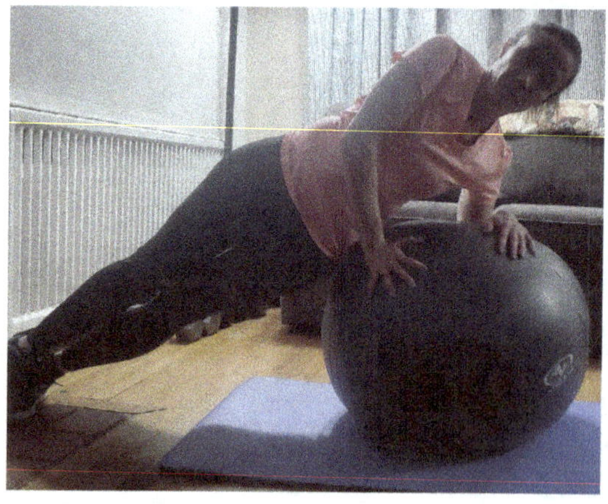

<u>30. Side Plank Hip Drops</u>
Intermediate

For this exercise, you will be in a side plank with the bottom hand on the floor directly underneath the shoulder. The stability ball will be between both feet and the body is in a straight line. The top hand can be extended straight up into the air or bent so the fingertips are at the temple. This is the starting position. Next you will lower the bottom hip by bending sideways at the waist. Return to the start position, stopping when the body has returned to a straight line. Don't reach the top hip up too high. This completes one rep. Repeat evenly on each side.

What it Works: The upper body, particularly the shoulders, need to work to support the body and the whole body must work to maintain balance, but this is primarily an oblique exercise.

Begin with 1 set of 5 reps, building to 3 sets of 10 reps.

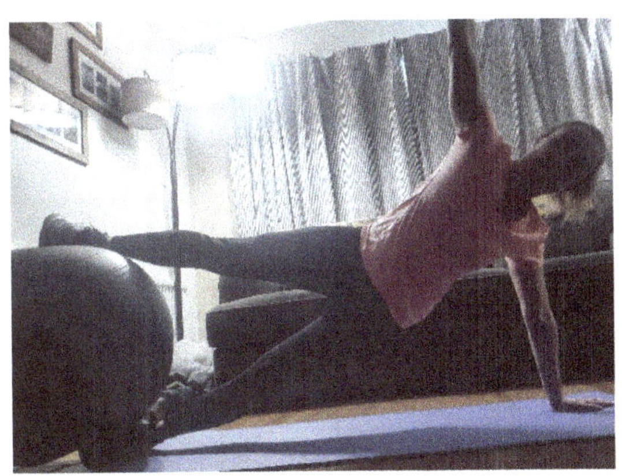

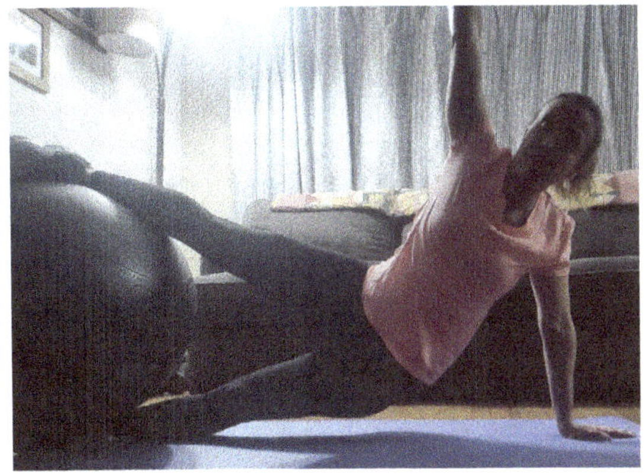

<u>31. Spidermans</u>
Intermediate

Begin this exercise by getting into a plank position with hands on the floor and the shins on the stability ball. Be careful not to arch the back and maintain the correct plank position with the tailbone tucked and wrists under shoulders. To perform this exercise you will bend one knee out to the side and pull it into the outside of the elbow. Return to the start position and repeat on the other side. This is one rep.

What it Works: This exercise primarily concentrates on the obliques and transverse abs.

Begin with 1 set of   10 reps, building
to 3 sets of 10 reps.

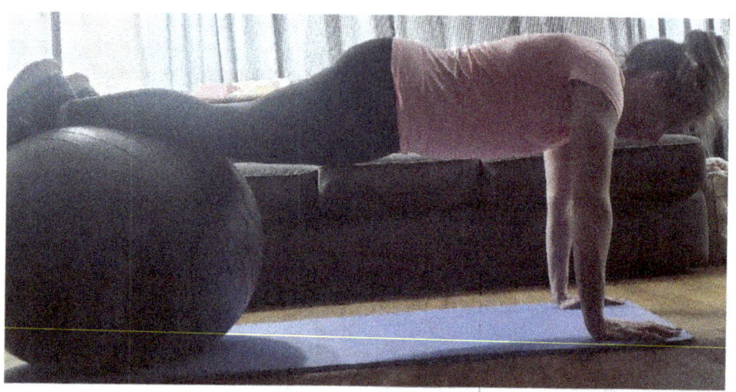

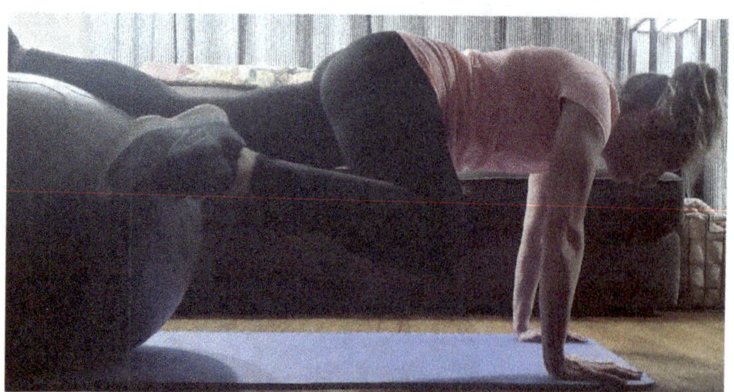

<u>32. Tucks</u>
Beginner-Intermediate

Begin this exercise by getting into a plank position with hands on the floor and the shins on the stability ball. Be careful not to arch the back and maintain the correct plank position with the tailbone tucked and wrists under shoulders. To perform this exercise you will bend the knees in towards the chin and roll the stability ball forward. Then rolling the ball back and returning to plank. This completes one rep.

What it Works: Planks are a total body exercise in which the core and shoulders must be engaged throughout. This exercise primarily focuses on the lower abdominal muscles.

Begin with 1 set of 5 reps, building to 3 sets of 5 reps, then 2 sets of 10 and finally 3 sets of 10 reps.

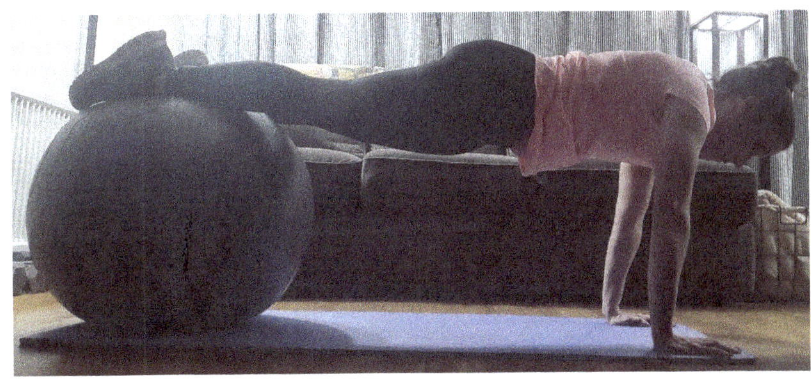

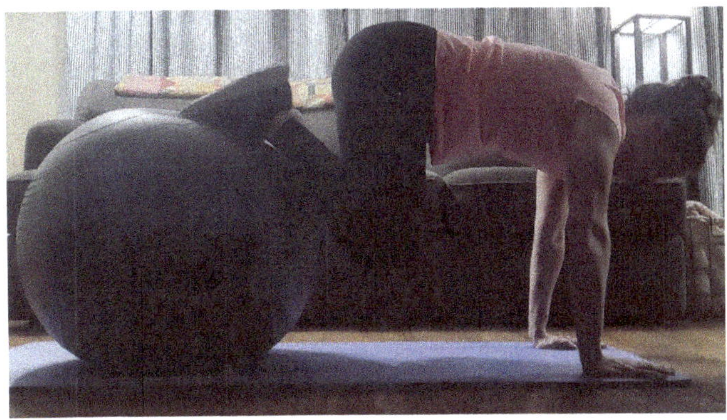

33. Pikes
Intermediate

Begin this exercise by getting into a plank position with hands on the floor and the shins on the stability ball. Be careful not to arch the back and maintain the correct plank position with the tailbone tucked and wrists under shoulders. Keeping the legs straight throughout, you will engage the core muscles and use them to roll the ball in towards the head and lifting the tailbone up creating an A shape. Lower back down to plank. This completes one rep.

What it Works: Planks are a total body exercise in which the core and shoulders must be engaged throughout. This exercise primarily focuses on the lower abdominal muscles.

Begin with 1 set of 5 reps, building to 3 sets of 5 reps, then 2 sets of 10 and finally 3 sets of 10 reps.

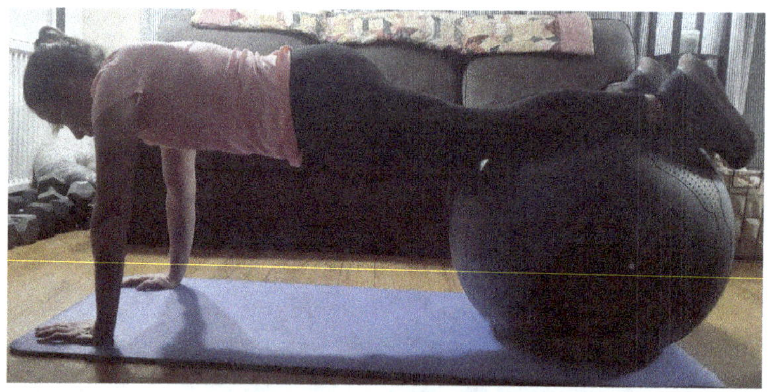

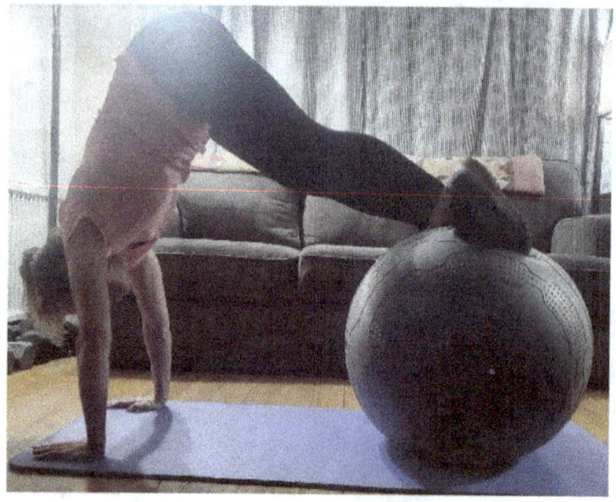

<u>34. Jackknife Twists</u>
Intermediate

Begin this exercise in a full plank position with hands on the floor and directly under the shoulders, body flat, tailbone tucked and tops of the feet on the stability ball. You will tuck the knees in diagonally towards the opposite shoulder, being careful to keep the upper body still throughout. Roll the stability ball back to the start and repeat on the other side. This completes one rep.

What it Works: This is a total body exercise as the core and shoulders must stay engaged throughout and the legs are working to pull the ball in. But this is primarily an abdominal exercise, specifically the rectus abdominis, transverse abdominis and obliques.

Begin with 1 set of 5 reps, building to 3 sets of 10 reps.

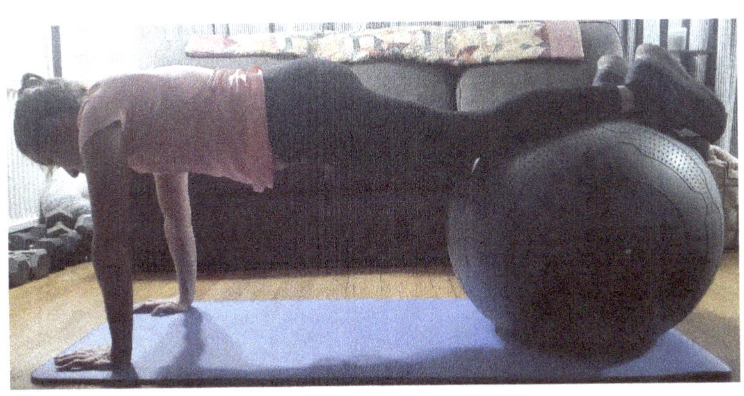

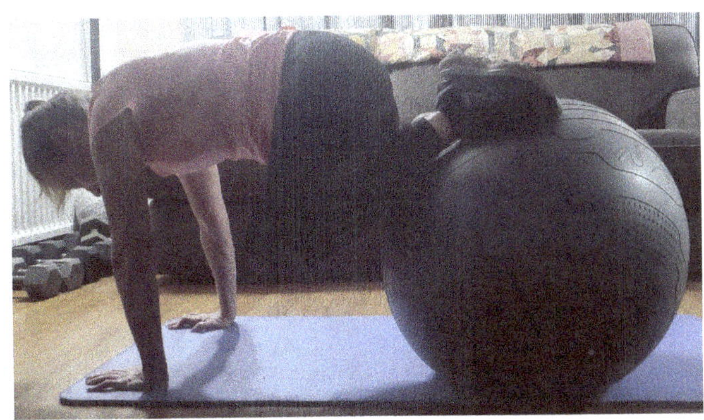

<u>35. Grasshoppers</u>
Intermediate-Advanced

Begin this exercise in a full plank position with hands on the floor and directly under the shoulders, body flat, tailbone tucked and tops of the feet on the stability ball.   First you will bring one knee in towards the chest, then you will extend that leg towards the opposite side of the stability ball by twisting at the waist. Return to the start position and repeat on the other side. This completes one rep.

What it Works: This is a total body exercise, but it primarily targets the lower (or transverse) abs as well as the obliques.

Begin with 1 set of 5 reps, building to 3 sets of 10 reps.

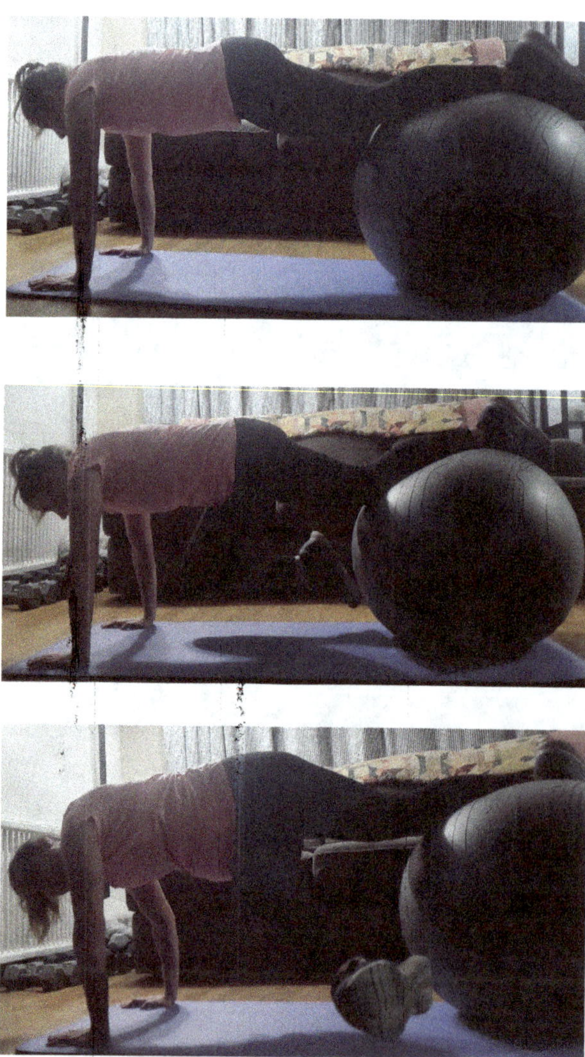

<u>36. Straight Legged Reverse Corkscrews</u>
Intermediate-Advanced

     Begin this exercise in a full plank position with the hands on the floor directly under the shoulders, the body is a straight line and the feet resting on top of the stability ball. To perform this exercise, you will extend one leg up and cross it over the other leg, touching the toes down on the opposite side of the ball before bringing it back to the start position. This completes one rep. Repeat evenly on each side.

What it Works: Although the total body is engaged and the back assists with this motion, this is primarily an abdominal exercise.

Begin with 1 set of 5 reps, building to 3 sets of 10 reps.

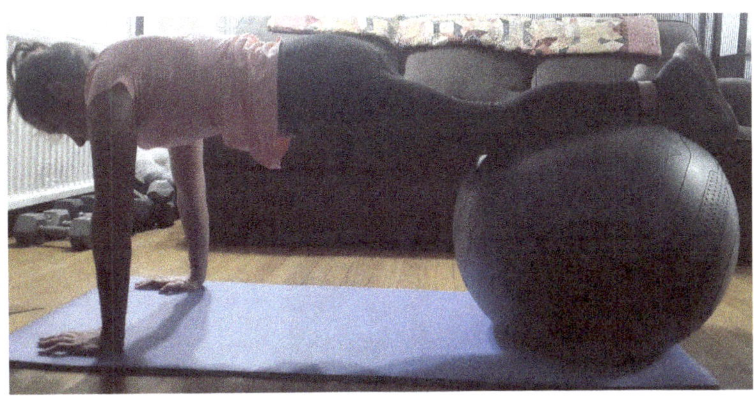

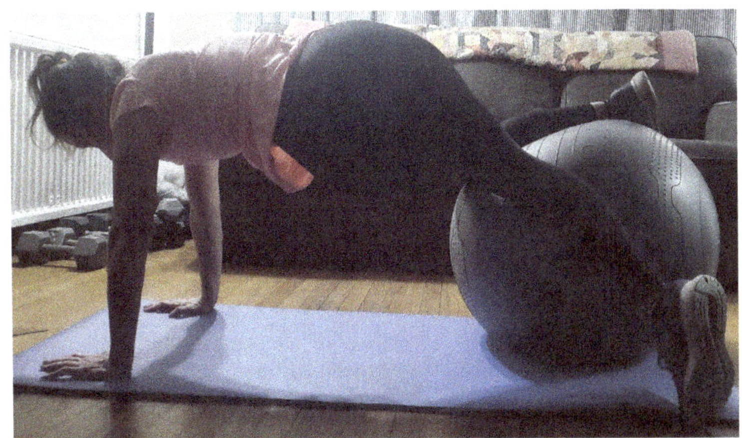

<u>37. Plank Jacks</u>
Beginner-Intermediate

Begin this exercise from a forearm plank position with the forearms resting on the stability ball. The elbows should be directly under the shoulders and the body should be in a straight line with the tailbone tucked. Feet are hip width apart and the balls of the feet are anchored to the floor. Keeping the hips and shoulders even throughout, you will jump the feet out to a wide stance then jump back to the start position. This completes on rep.

What it Works: Planks are a total body exercise, but this primarily focuses on the lower or transverse abs.

Begin with 1 set of 5 reps, building to 3 sets of 10 reps.

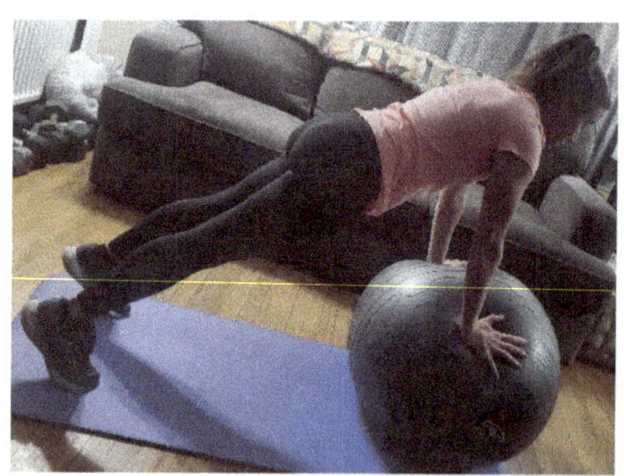

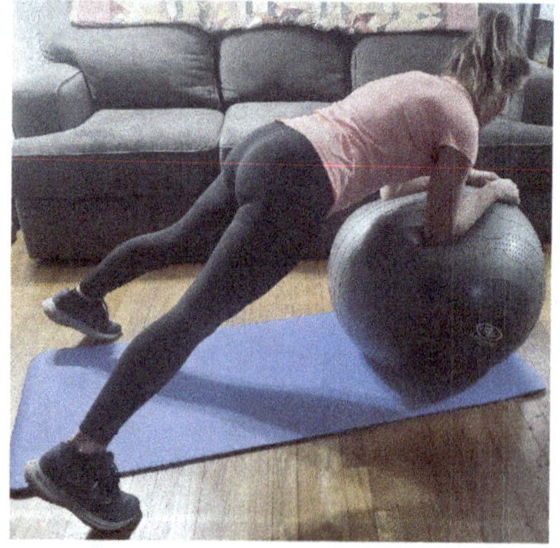

<u>38. Mountain Climbers</u>
Beginner-Intermediate

You will be in a full plank throughout this exercise with hands on the stability ball and shoulders above the wrists. (Can be modified by doing a hover plank instead.) Toes will be anchored to the floor and the body will be in a straight line from head to heels. To perform this exercise you will first bring one knee in to touch the stability ball while driving the opposite foot back and into the floor. Hop your legs into the opposite position to complete the exercise on the other side. This completes one rep.

What it Works: This is a total body exercise as the shoulders must support and balance and the legs must support and drive forward, but it is primarily a core exercise. Specifically the lower abdominals and obliques.

Begin with 1 set of 5 reps, building to 3 sets of 15 reps.

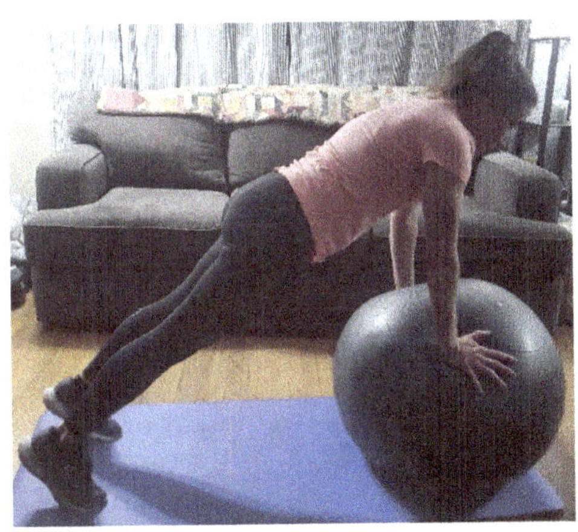

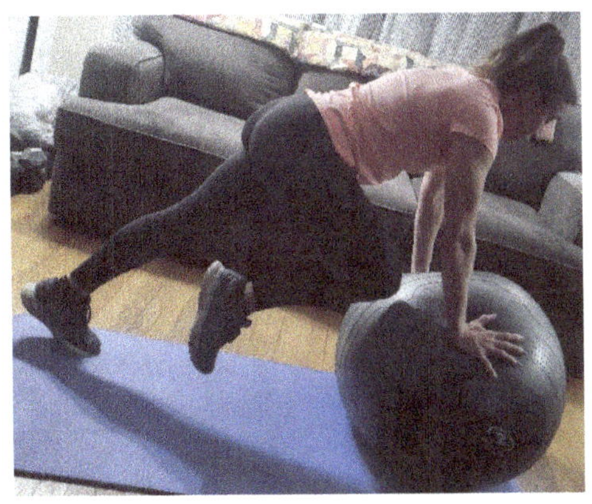

<u>39. Plank Crossovers</u>
Beginner-Intermediate

You will be in a full plank throughout this exercise with hands on the stability ball and shoulders above the wrists. (Can be modified by doing a hover plank instead). Toes will be anchored to the floor and the body will be in a straight line from head to heels. To perform this exercise you will first bring one knee across the body to touch the stability ball under the opposite arm while driving the opposite foot back and into the floor. Hop your legs into the opposite position to complete the exercise on the other side. This completes one rep.

What it Works: This is a total body exercise as the shoulders must support and balance and the legs must support and drive forward, but it is primarily a core exercise. Specifically the lower abdominals and obliques.

Begin with 1 set of 5 reps, building to 3 sets of 15 reps.

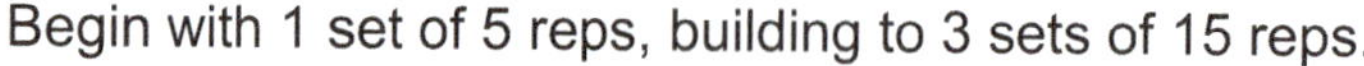

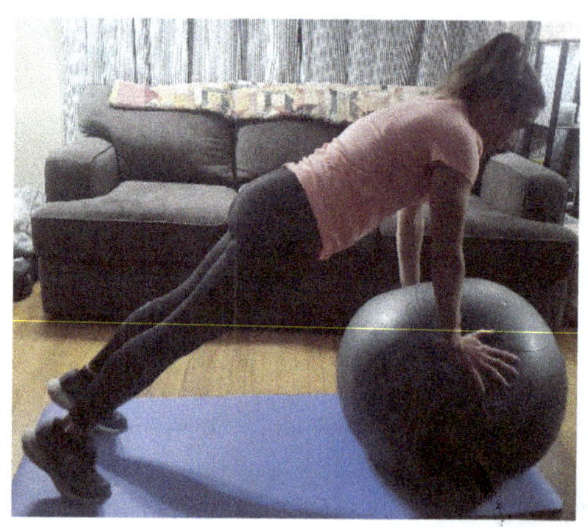

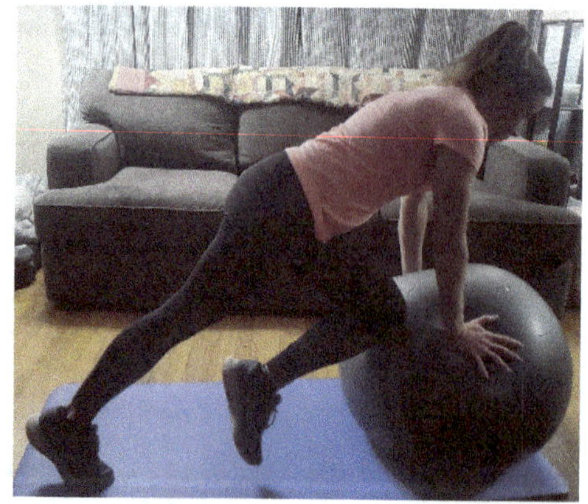

<u>40. Table Top Planks</u>
Beginner-Intermediate

From a kneeling position with toes pressed into the floor, lean forward and rest the elbows and forearms on the stability ball. The body should be a straight line from the head down to the knees, careful not to arch the back. To perform this exercise, raise the knees off the floor and straighten the legs out while staying on the forearms on the stability ball. The body should now be a straight line from the head down to the feet. Hold for 3 seconds and lower back down to start. This is one rep.

What it Works: This exercise focuses on the muscles of the core. Predominantly the abdominals as well as the glutes.

Begin with 1 set of 5 reps, building to 3 sets of 5 reps. Ultimately building up to 3 sets of 15 reps.

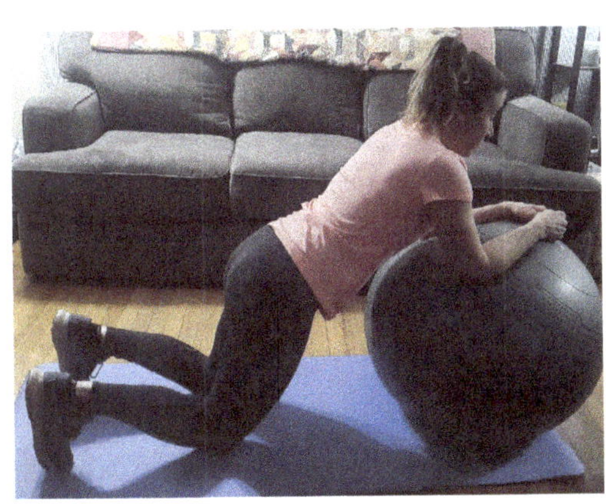

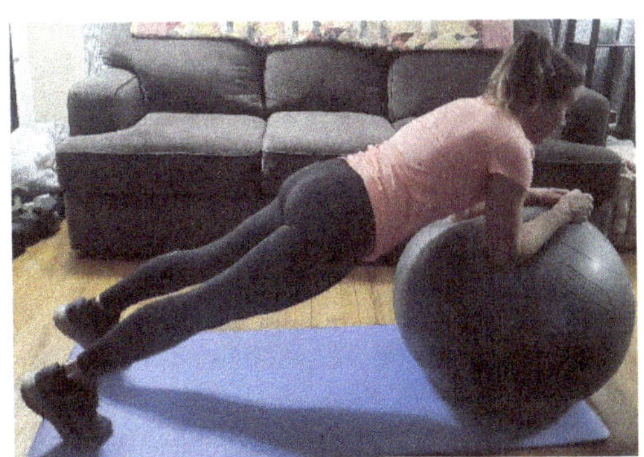

<u>41. Ab Rollout</u>
Intermediate

Begin this exercise from a kneeling position with the torso stretched up tall and arms extended straight, resting clenched fists on top of the stability ball. To perform this exercise, you will lean the body forward while maintaining a straight line from the knees to the head by allowing the ball to roll down to the forearms and stopping once the ball has reached the elbows. Be careful to maintain a straight back throughout. Push the body back upright by contracting the abdominals. This completes one rep.

What it Works: Although the chest and shoulders are engaged, this is primarily an abdominal exercise.

Begin with 1 set of 5 reps, building to 3 sets of 5 reps, then 2 sets of 10 and finally 3 sets of 10 reps.

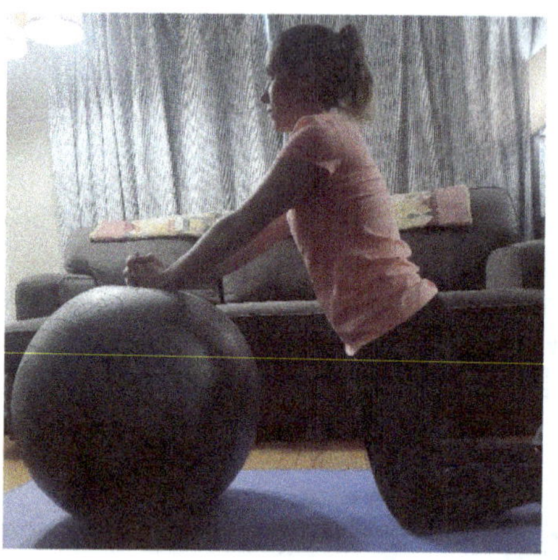

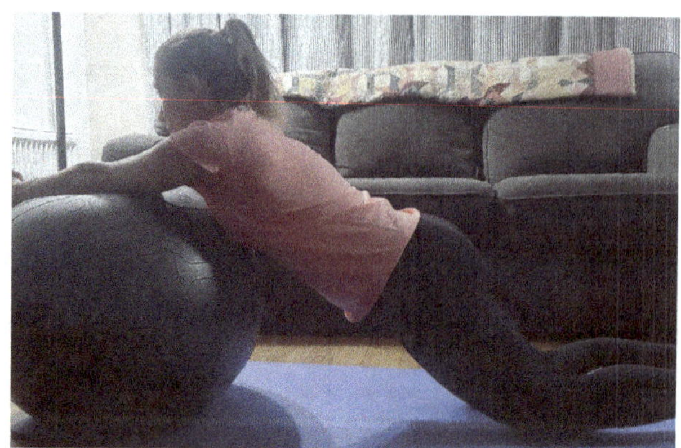

<u>42. Plank Rollout</u>
Advanced

Begin this exercise in a forearm plank with the forearms on the stability ball, the elbows under the shoulders, body in a straight line with the tailbone tucked and the balls of the feet anchored to the floor. To perform this exercise you will push the elbows forward, pause then pull back to the start position being careful to keep the back and hips straight throughout. This completes one rep.

What it Works: This exercise primarily targets the lower back and ab muscles (transverse and rectus abdominis.)

Begin with 1 set of 5 reps, building up to 3 sets of 10 reps.

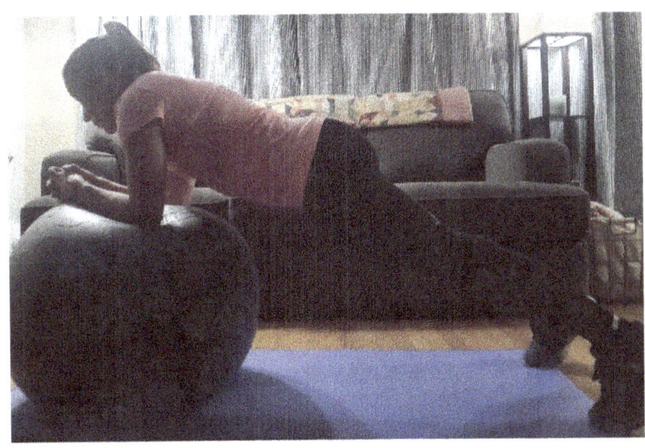

<u>43. Standing Ab Rollout</u>
Intermediate

From a standing position in a very wide stance, roll the body forward while tucking the tailbone and bracing the core. The hands can be clasped together as one fist and will be resting on top of the stability ball. To perform this exercise, you will roll forward across your forearms stopping once the elbow has reached the stability ball and the body is in a straight line. Return to the start position.

What it Works: This is an advanced exercise that targets the abdominal muscles.

Begin with 1 set of 3 reps, building to 3 sets of 10 reps.

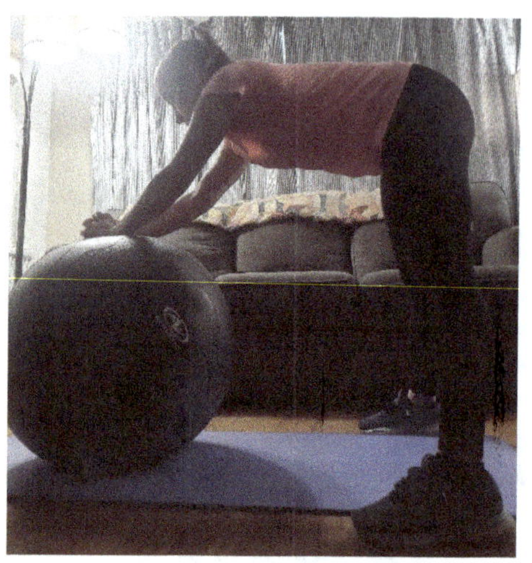

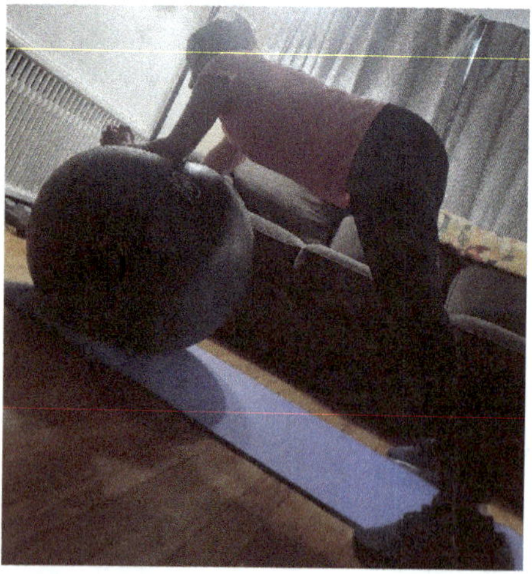

<u>44. Stir the Pot</u>
Intermediate-Advanced

Start in the kneeling plank position with the knees anchored to the floor, body angled in a straight line with tailbone tucked , back straight and elbows resting on the stability ball underneath the shoulders. The body should be in a straight line from head to knees. Roll the stability ball by moving the forearms in a clockwise motion. The rest of the body will remain still and only the arms will be moving the stability ball. Repeat evenly on each side by rolling the ball in a counterclockwise motion. One full rotation completes one rep.

What it Works: Although the arms and core will be engaged throughout this exercise, it primarily focuses on the abs.

Begin with 1 set of 5 reps, building to 3 sets of 5 reps, then 2 sets of 10 and finally 3 sets of 10 reps.

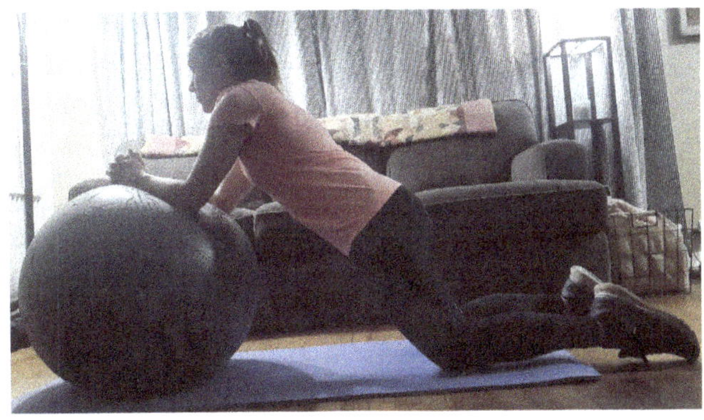

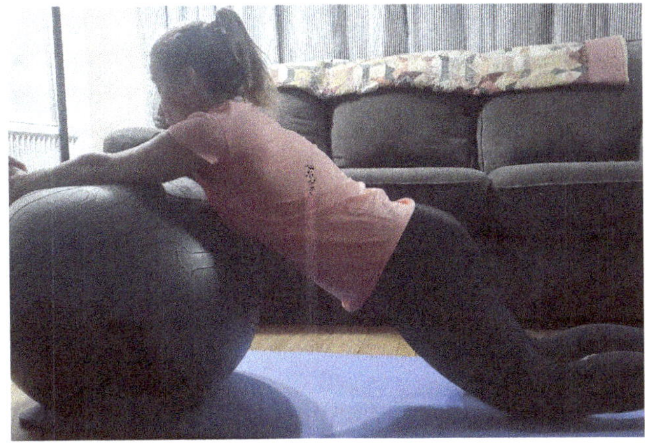

<u>45. Arm and Leg Extension Reaches</u>
Beginner-Intermediate

From a full plank with hands under shoulders, body straight and toes anchored into the floor, position the stability ball under the hips. The body should stay stable and level throughout. To perform this exercise, you will extend one arm forward while raising the opposite leg straight up. Repeat on the opposite arm and leg. This completes one rep.

What it Works: This is a total body exercise. The legs and shoulders are doing some work, but the majority of the work is actually in the core (primarily the back) as it stabilizes the body through this motion.

Begin with 1 set of 5 reps, building to 3 sets of 5 reps, then 2 sets of 10 and finally 3 sets of 10 reps.

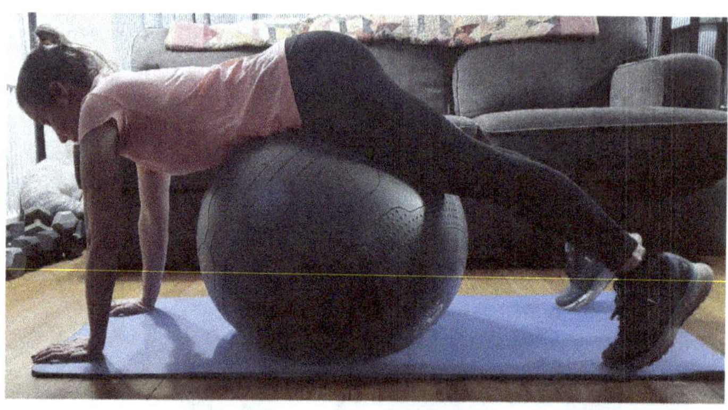

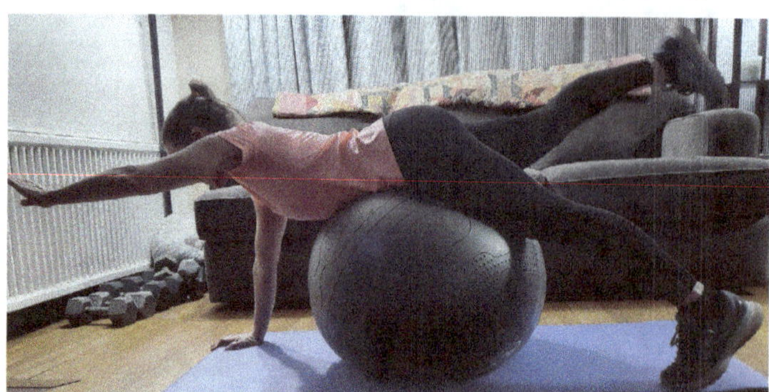

46. Cobra
Beginner-Intermediate

Begin by lying face down, legs extended out straight and the stability ball between both hands with arms stretched out straight overhead. The lower body will remain anchored to the floor throughout. To perform this exercise, you will raise the stability ball up off the floor by lifting the chest up off the floor. Lower back down to the start. This completes one rep.

What it Works: This exercise primarily targets the muscle the runs along the spine, called the erector spinae.

Begin with 1 set of 5 reps, building to 3 sets of 5 reps, then 2 sets of 10 and finally 3 sets of 10 reps.

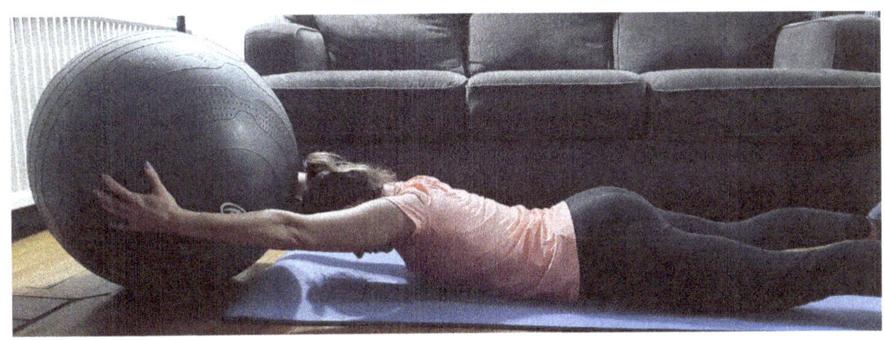

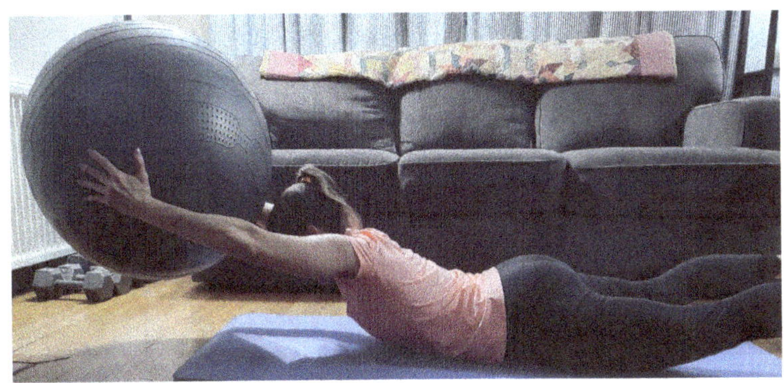

<u>47. Superman with Arm Pull Back</u>
Beginner-Intermediate

Lying face down on the floor, the stability ball should be positioned between both feet with legs extended straight out behind. With arms extended straight overhead, you will perform this exercise by bringing the upper and lower body off the floor at the same time so the limbs are hovering. Raise the chest up and pull one elbow back and in towards the body and lower back down. Repeat on the other side. This completes one rep.

What it Works: This is a total body exercise that mainly concentrates on the muscles of the back.

Begin with 1 set of 5 reps, building to 3 sets of 5 reps, then 2 sets of 10 and finally 3 sets of 10 reps.

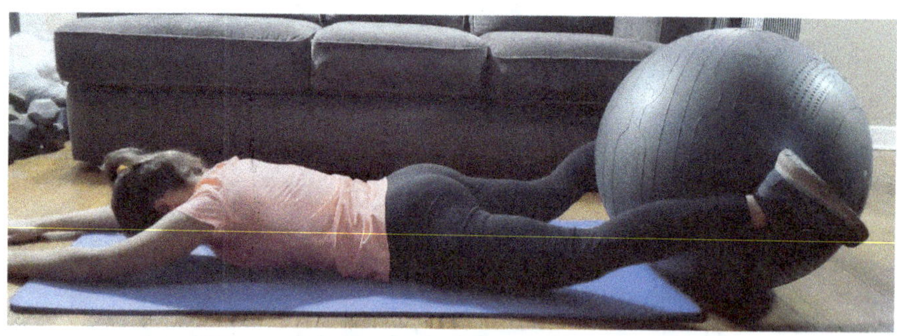

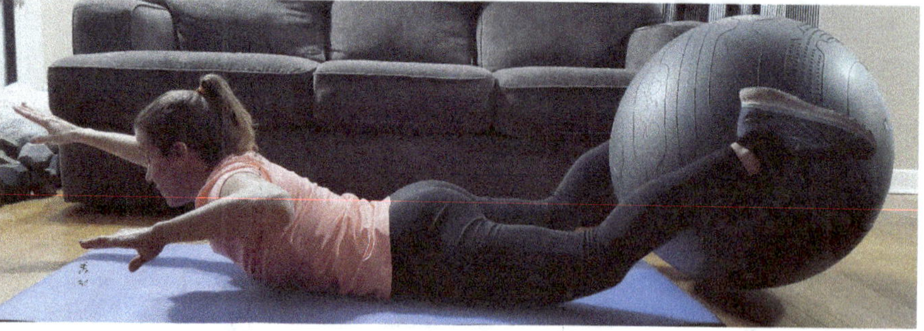

<u>48. Back Extension</u>
Beginner-Intermediate

Lie face down with hips on the stability ball and legs extended straight behind with toes planted on the floor. Place the fingertips at the temples with elbows bent out wide. The torso will be relaxed over the ball. To perform this exercise, you will raise the chest up creating a straight line from the head down to the feet. Hold for 3 seconds at the top before lowering back down. This is one rep.

What it Works: Primarily focuses on the muscle that runs along the spine (the erector spinae).

Begin with 1 set of 5 reps, building to 3 sets of 5 reps, then 2 sets of 10 and finally 3 sets of 10 reps.

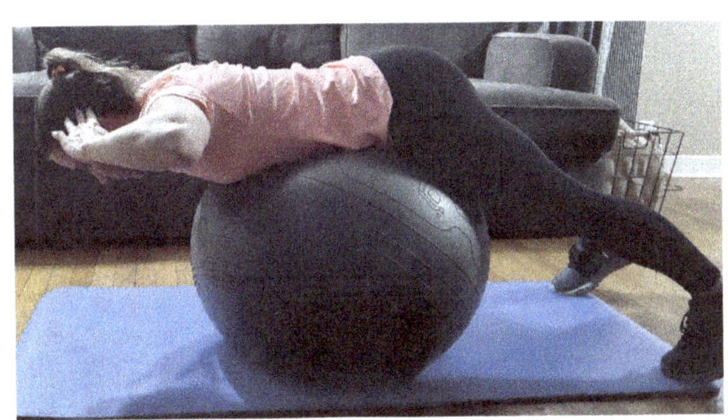

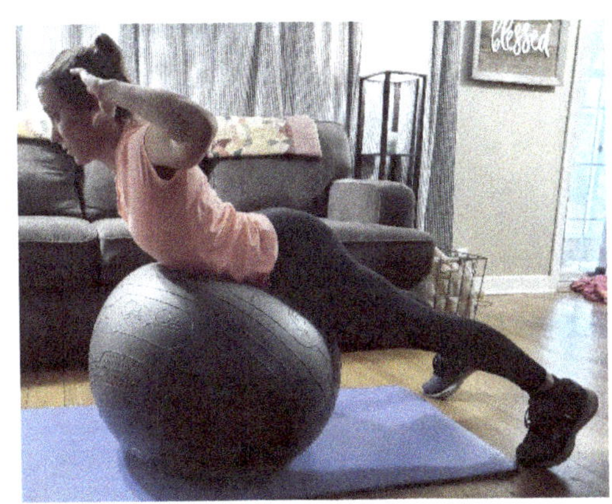

<u>49. Prone Cobra</u>
Beginner

Lie face down so that the midsection is resting on top of the stability ball. The body should be in a straight line with the toes anchored to the floor and the arms stretched out overhead. To perform this exercise, you will keep your arms stretched out straight and bring them behind you, keeping the palms facing down throughout. Return to the start position. This completes one rep.

What it Works: Although the shoulders will be engaged, this is primarily an exercise that targets the muscles of the mid and lower back.

Begin with 1 set of 10 reps, building to 3 sets of 15 reps.

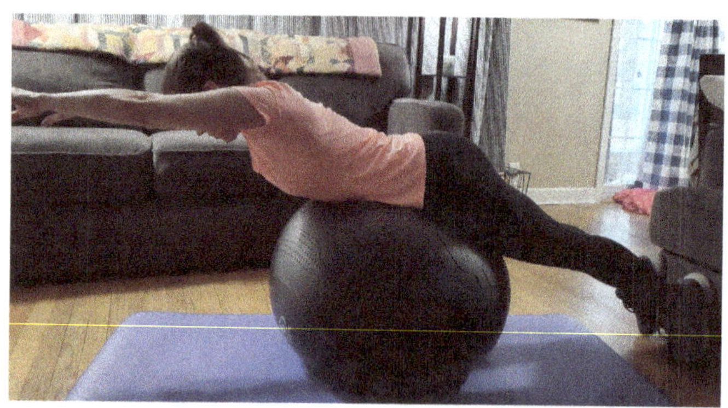

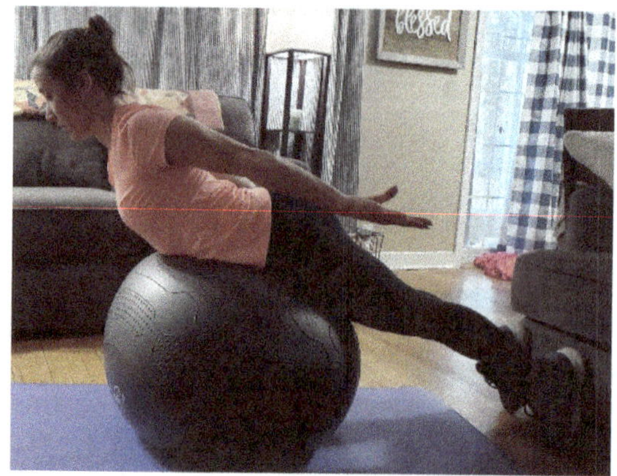

<u>50. Back Extension with a Twist</u>
Beginner-Intermediate

Lie face down with hips on the stability ball and legs extended straight behind with toes planted on the floor. Place the fingertips at the temples with elbows bent out wide. The torso will be relaxed over the ball. To perform this exercise, you will raise the chest up creating a straight line from the head down to the feet. At the top, you will rotate the torso to the side by twisting towards the side wall. Lower back to the start position and repeat on the other side. This completes one rep.

What it Works: This exercise engages the core, primarily focusing on the muscle that runs along the spine (the erector spinae).

Begin with 1 set of 5 reps, building to 3 sets of 5 reps, then 2 sets of 10 and finally 3 sets of 10 reps.

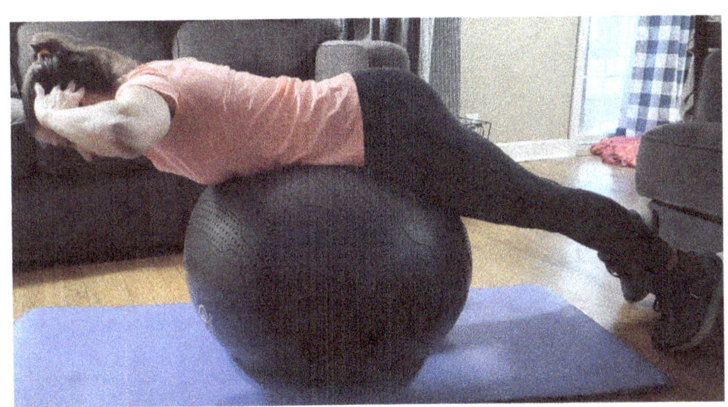

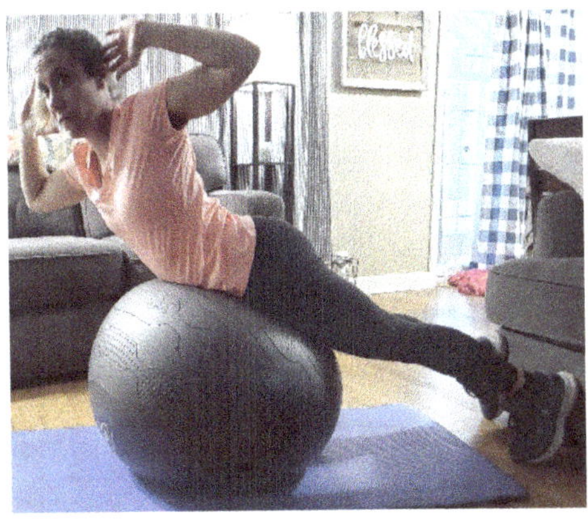

<u>51. Boat Bose Pull Down</u>
Beginner-Intermediate

Starting from a seated position, lean the torso back at a 45 degree angle and lift the legs off the ground to hover while keeping them extended out straight. Holding the stability ball in both hands, reach the arms up straight overhead. This is the starting position. While maintaining the boat pose with the body throughout, you will bend the arms lowering the stability ball behind the head. Return to the start position. That makes one rep.

What it Works: This exercise engages the core throughout as the abs must be contracted to hold the boat pose, but the muscles of the shoulders and upper back are the main focus.

Begin with 1 set of 5 reps, building to 3 sets of 10 reps.

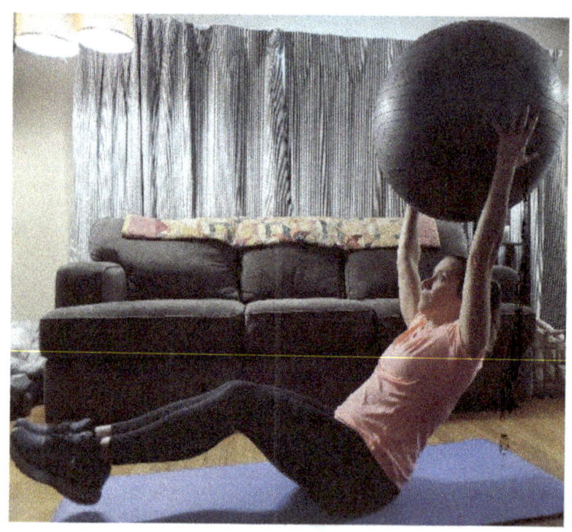

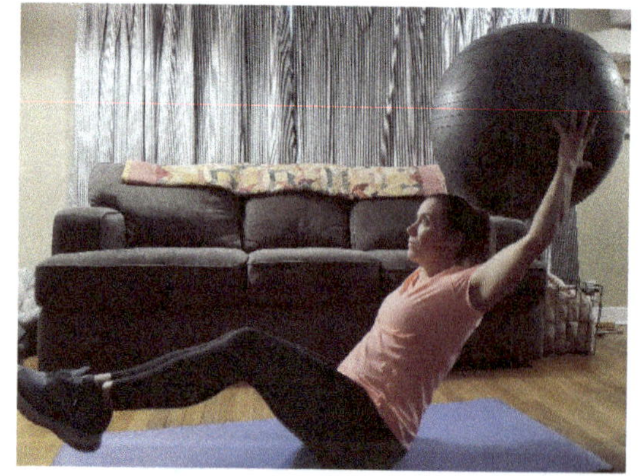

<u>52. Kneeling Lat Pull</u>
Beginner

Begin this exercise by kneeling with the butt resting on the heels. Rest the forearms on the stability ball in front of you, with arms straight and palms facing towards each other but not touching. Roll the ball forward so the tailbone drives back and down and the torso folds forward so the face is down. To perform this exercise, you will roll the stability ball back while keeping the arms straight and allowing the hips to rise as well as the torso so the body is now in an upright kneel. Roll the ball back forward to the starting position. This completes one rep.

What it Works: This exercise primarily concentrates on the muscles of the upper back.

Begin with 1 set of 10 reps, building to as many as 3 sets of 15 reps.

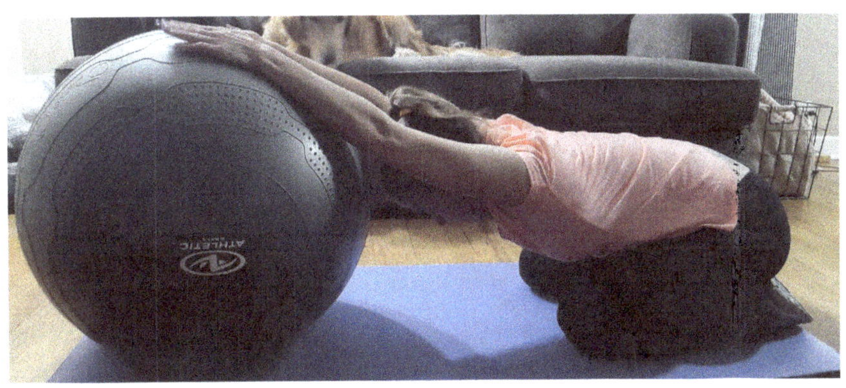

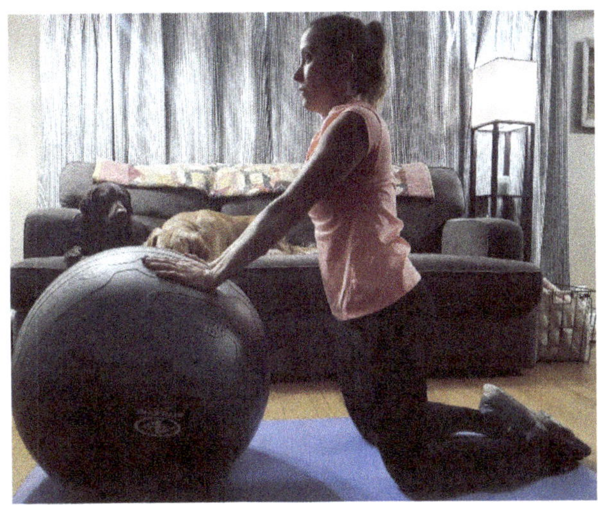

<u>53. Kneeling Tricep Extension</u>
Beginner

From a kneeling position with your butt resting on your heels, you will rest the stability ball on your lap. Extend the arms out straight so the elbows and forearms are resting on the stability ball. To perform this exercise, you will bend the elbows at 90 degrees and raise the forearms so they are pointing straight up and the elbows are driving down into the ball. Return to the start position. This completes one rep.

What it Works: This exercise focuses on the muscles on the backside of the upper arm, or the triceps muscle.

Begin with 1 set of 10 reps, building to 3 sets of 10 reps.

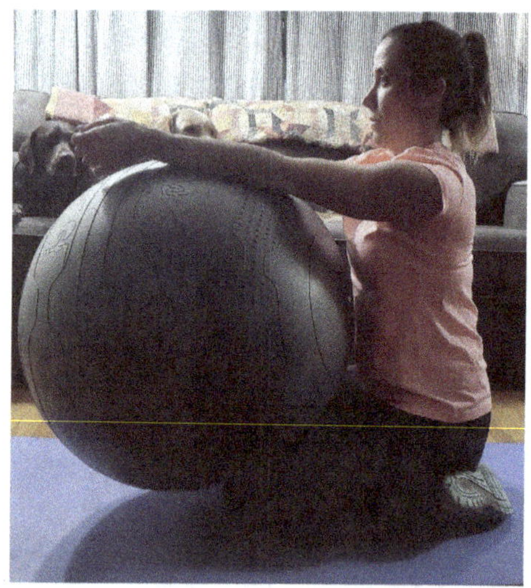

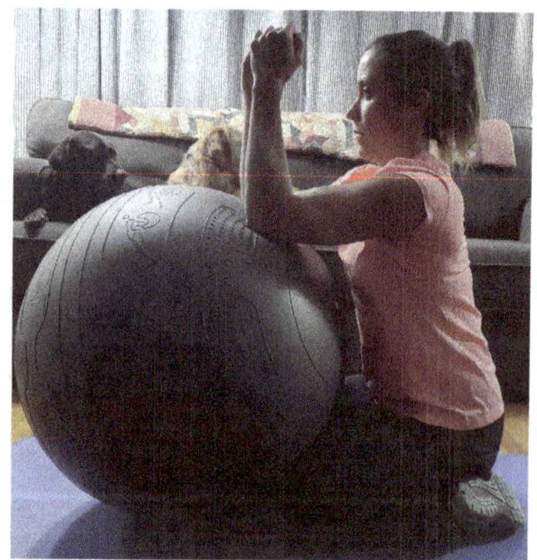

<u>54. Triceps Dips</u>
Advanced

For this exercise, it is a good idea to put the stability ball in a corner or against a wall. You will sit on the stability ball with your hands on either side of you with the fingertips pointing forward. Walk your feet out so that only the palms are on the ball supporting the body along with the heels. Bending the elbows straight back, you will lower your butt down and away from the ball, stopping before you hit the floor. Push yourself back up to the start position. This completes one rep.

What it Works: This exercise primarily targets the triceps muscles on the back side of the upper arm.

Begin with 1 set of 5 reps, building to 3 sets of 10 reps.

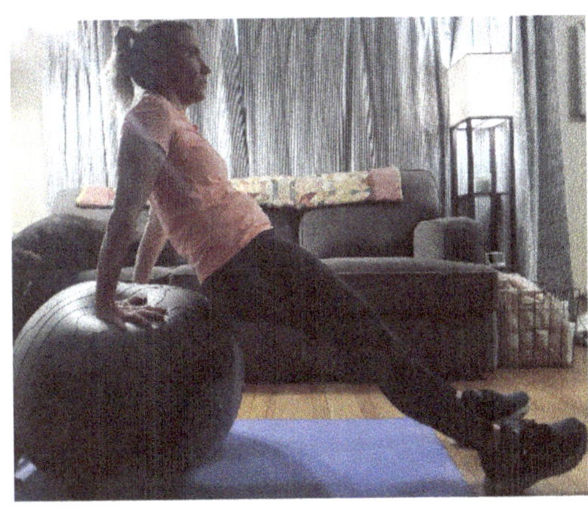

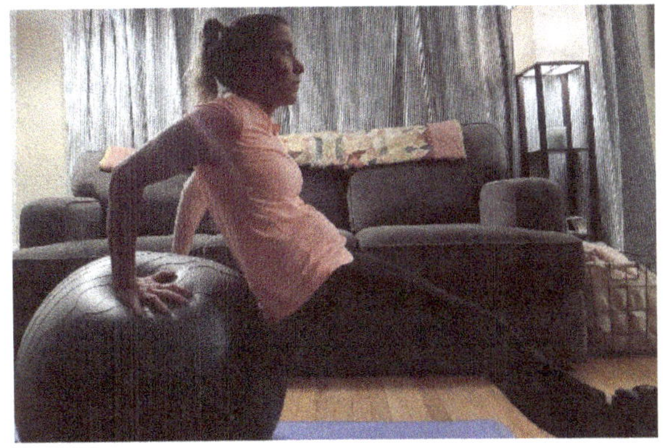

<u>55. Tricep Push-Ups</u>
Intermediate-Advanced

Begin in a full plank with the hands on the floor directly under the shoulders and the tops of the legs on top of the stability ball. Your body should be in a straight line. To perform this exercise, you will lower down into a tricep push up by dropping the chest down and bringing the elbows straight back. The arms should stay against the body as you lower and push yourself back to the start position by contracting your triceps. This completes one rep.

What it Works: Although the core must be engaged throughout and the shoulders are assisting, this is primarily a triceps exercise, which are the muscles on the backside of the upper arm.

Begin with 1 set of 5 reps, building to 3 sets of 10 reps.

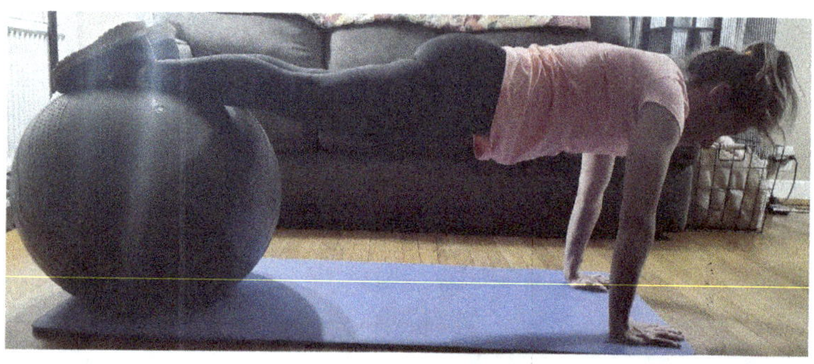

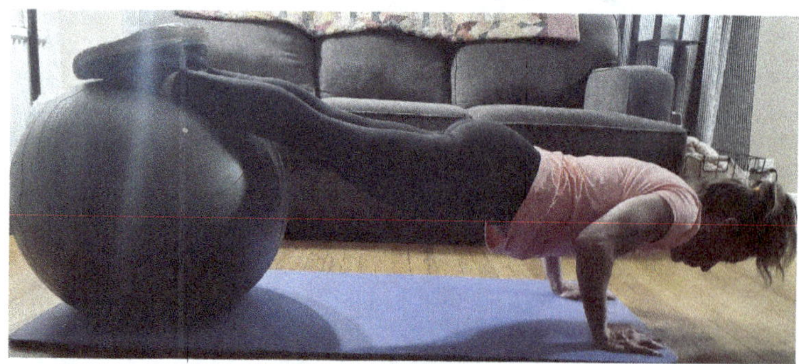

<u>56. Biceps Squeeze</u>
Beginner

From a kneeling position with butt resting on the heels, hold the stability ball out straight in front of your chest. To perform this exercise, you will bend the elbows, curling the ball up. Squeeze the biceps and hold for 3 seconds at the top before releasing back down. This is one rep.

What it Works: This exercise targets the muscle on the front of the upper arm, or the biceps.

Begin with 1 set of 10 reps, building to 3 sets of 10 reps.

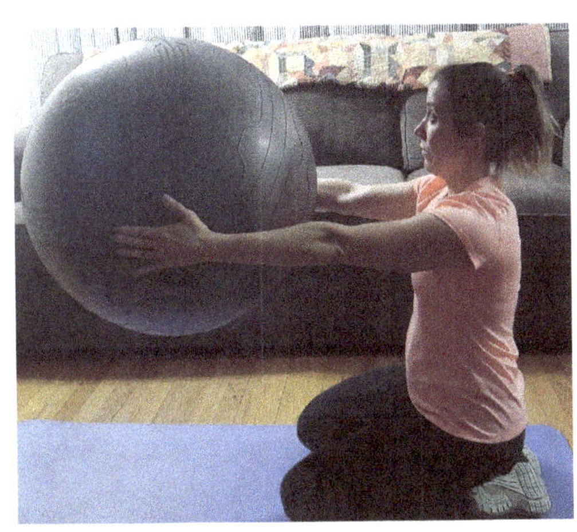

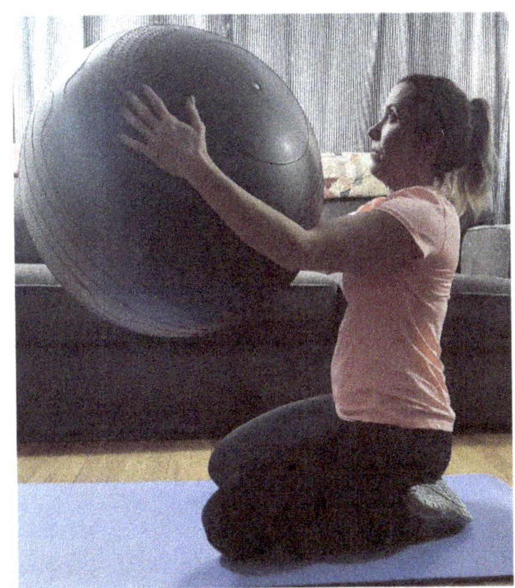

<u>57. Biceps Wall Curl</u>
Beginner

For this exercise, you will be in a standing position. The palms will be turned so the palms are against the stability ball and the ball will be at waist height and pressed between the palms and the wall. Keeping the body straight, you will step back so the body is at a slight incline leaning in towards the stability ball. Lift the heels up so you are balancing on your toes. This is the start position. To perform this exercise you will lean in while curling the biceps up and rolling the ball up the wall until the forearms are parallel to the floor. Roll back down to the start position. This is one rep.

What it Works: This exercise primarily targets the biceps, although the legs are working as well.

Begin with 1 set of 10 reps, building to 3 sets of 10 reps.

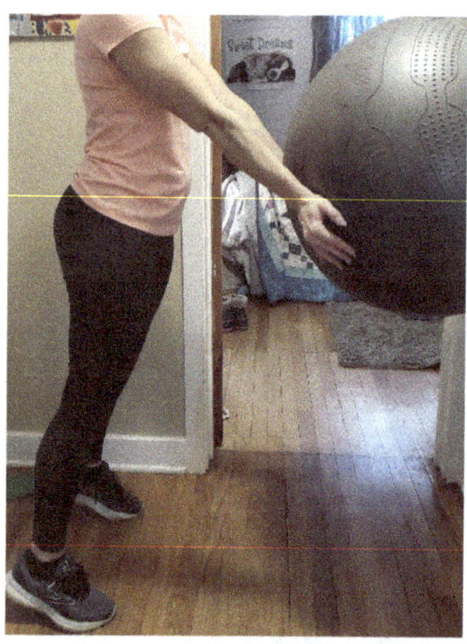 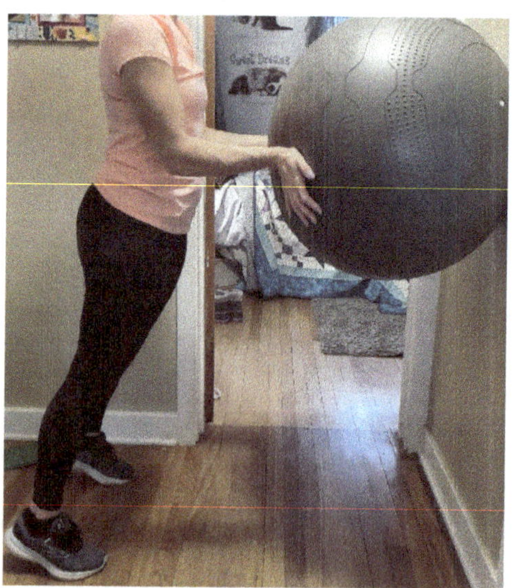

<u>58. Shoulder Roll</u>
Beginner

From a kneeling position, rest the butt back onto the heels and hold the stability ball in both hands with arms extended out in front of the chest. To perform this exercise, you will rotate the shoulders in circles by rolling them forwards and backwards, keeping the arms stretched out straight throughout. One full rotation is one rep.

What it Works: This exercise concentrates on the muscles of the shoulders.

Begin with 1 set of 10 reps, building to 3 sets of 10 reps.

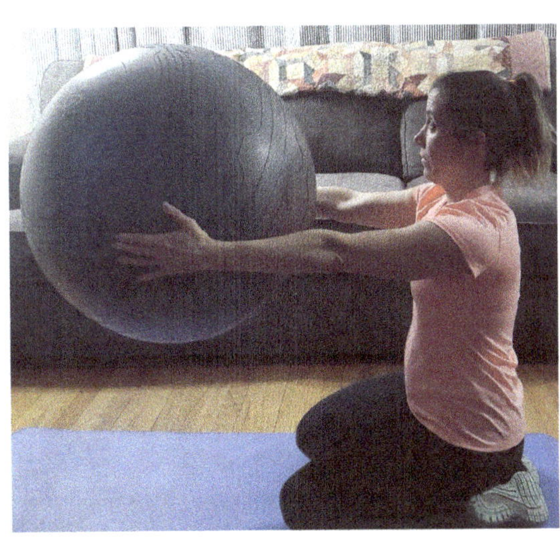

<u>59. I-Y-T Shoulder Raise</u>
Beginner

Lie face down on the stability ball with your hips and abdomen on the ball, legs stretched out straight behind you with toes pressed into the floor.   Your body should be in a straight line from head to feet throughout. Allow the arms to hang with clenched fists making 'thumbs up.' This is the starting position. To perform this exercise, you will first raise the arms straight up overhead making an "I" then lower back down to start. Next raise the arms up at a diagonal overhead making a "Y" then lower back down. Last you will raise the arms out to the side making a "T" before lowering back to start. This is one rep.

What it Works: Although the core must be engaged throughout in order to maintain a straight line, this predominantly works the back and shoulder muscles.

Begin 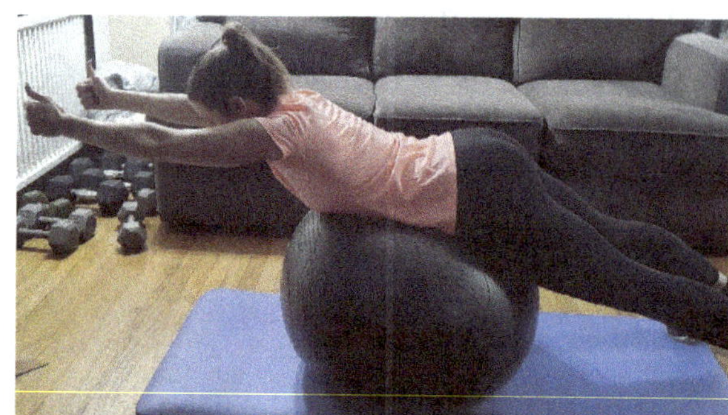 with 1 set of 5 reps, building to 3 sets of
15 reps.

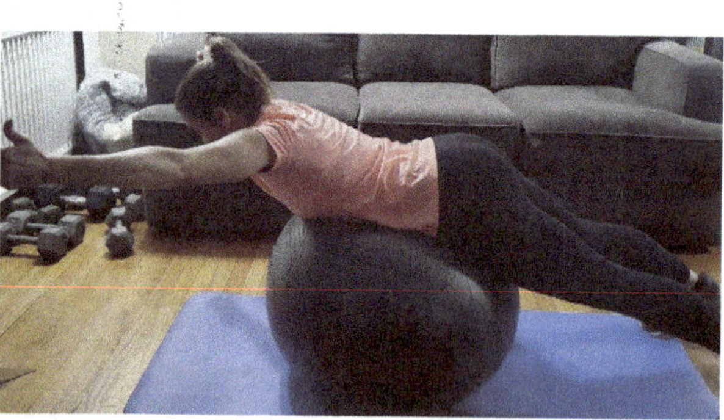

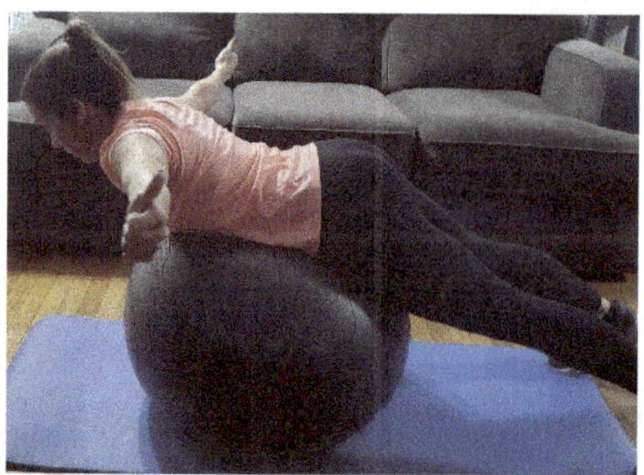

<u>60. Pec Squeeze</u>
Beginner

From a kneeling position with your butt resting on your heels, you will hug the stability ball in front of your chest using your hands and forearms with the arms softly bent. To perform this exercise, you will squeeze the ball in with your forearms and hold for 3 seconds before releasing. This is one rep.

What it Works: This exercise targets the muscles of the chest, or pecs.

Begin with 1 set of 5 reps, building to 3 sets of 10 reps.

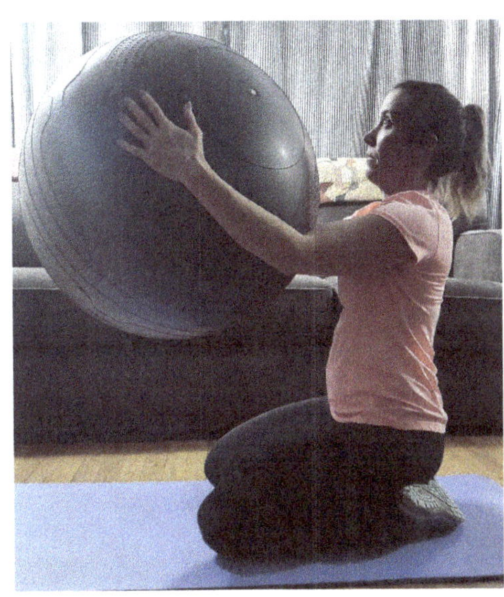

<u>61. Hollow Body Ball Toss</u>
Beginner-Intermediate

Begin by lying on your back with legs stretched out straight and the stability ball in both hands above the chest. Contract the abs as you bring the legs and head up to hover above the floor in a hollow body position. You will hold this position throughout as you toss the stability ball straight up. Each catch of the ball is one rep.

What it Works: The abs must be engaged throughout this entire exercise, but it is primarily working the chest and shoulders.

Begin with 1 set of 10 reps, building to 3 sets of 15 reps.

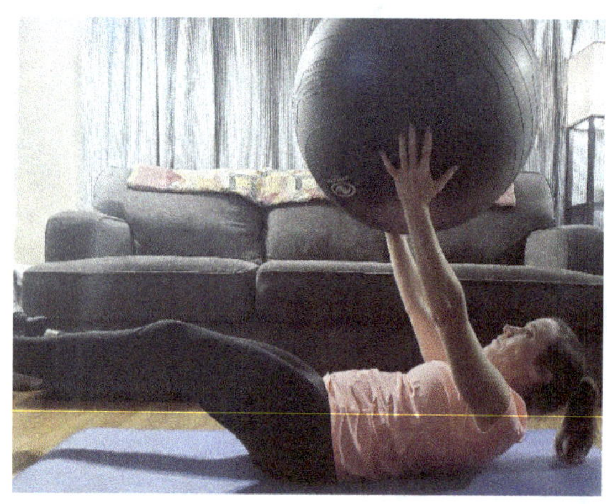

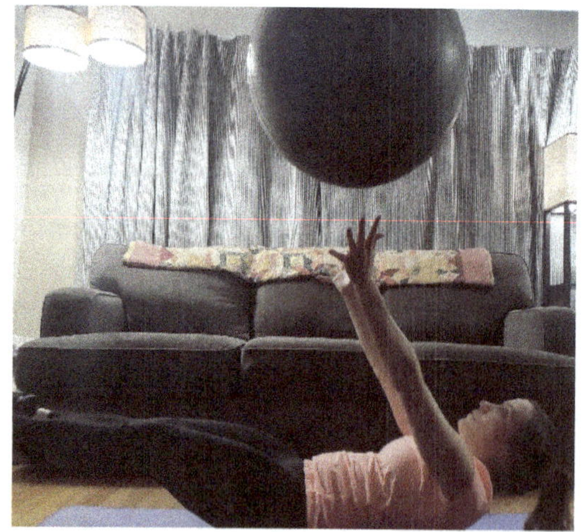

<u>62. Wall Push-Ups</u>
Beginner

From a standing position, extend the arms out straight in front of the chest and place the palms on the stability ball sandwiching it between the wall and your hands. Walk the feet back so you are leaned into the ball. The arms are still straight, the body is in a straight line and the toes are anchored into the floor. To perform this exercise, you will bend the arms, lowering the chest to elbow height. Push back up to the start position. This completes one rep.

What it Works: This exercise targets the muscles of the chest, although the shoulders and core are also engaged.

Begin with 1 set of 10 reps, building up to 3 sets of 15 reps.

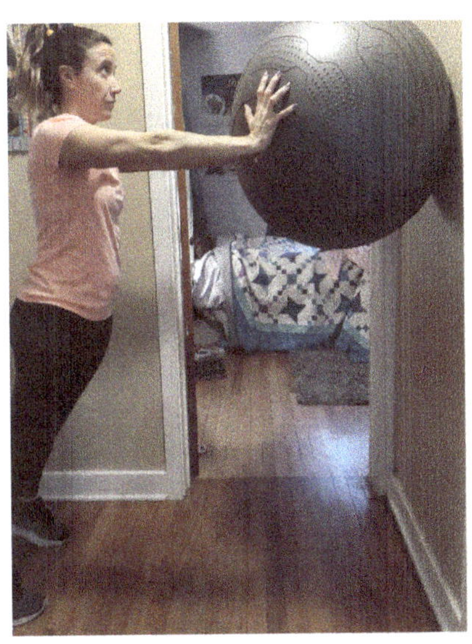
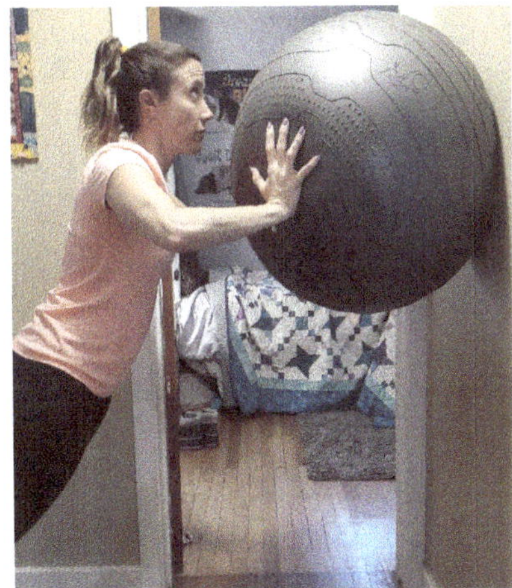

<u>63. Plank Shoulder Taps</u>
Intermediate-Advanced

For this exercise, you will be in a plank position with hands on the floor and shoulders directly above the wrists, the body will be in a straight line with a flat back and tailbone tucked while the tops of the feet rest on the stability ball. You will bend one arm and tap the opposite shoulder while being careful to keep the body even throughout. Repeat with the other hand. This completes one rep.

What it Works: The core must be engaged throughout this exercise, but the muscles of the chest and shoulders are the main workers.

Begin with 1 set of 5 reps, building to 3 sets of 10 reps.

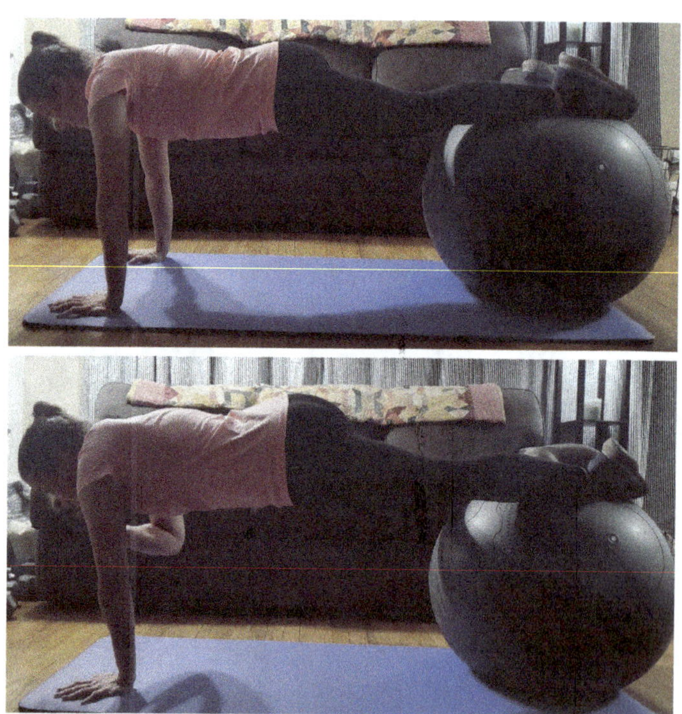

<u>64. Up Down Planks</u>
Intermediate

For this exercise, you will be in a plank position with hands on the floor and shoulders directly
above the wrists, the body will be in a straight line with a flat back and tailbone tucked while the
tops of the feet rest on the stability ball. You will lower down onto the forearms one arm at a
time, then return to the start position one arm at a time. Repeat with the opposite arm leading.
This completes one rep.

What it Works: This is a total body exercise as the core must be engaged throughout, but the
muscles of the chest and shoulders are the main workers.

Begin with 1 set of 5 reps, building to 4 sets of 10 reps.

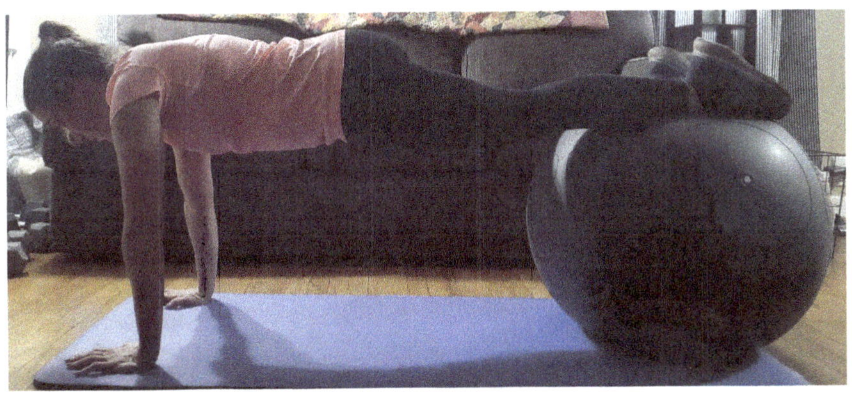

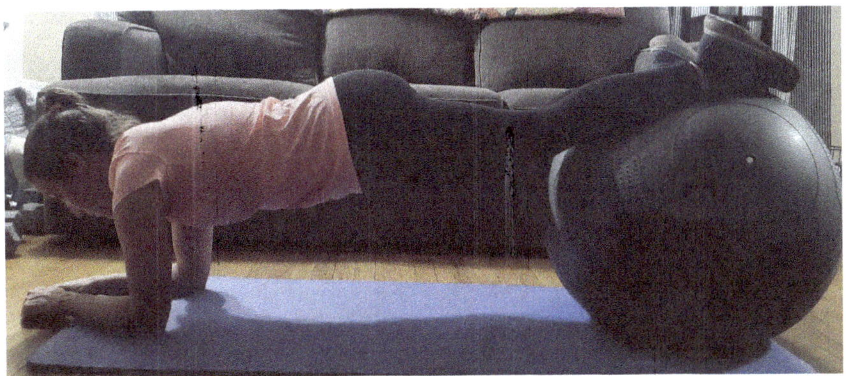

<u>65. Decline Push-Ups</u>
Intermediate

For this exercise, you will be in a plank position with hands on the floor and shoulders directly above the wrists, the body will be in a straight line with a flat back and tailbone tucked while the toes are pressed into the stability ball. To perform this exercise you will bend your elbows to lower your chest towards the floor. The elbows should stay tucked in close towards the body. Push your body back up to the start position. This completes one rep.

What it Works: This is a total body exercise, but the majority of the workload is on both the chest, arms and shoulders as well as the core as it maintains the proper plank form throughout.

Begin with 1 set of 5 reps, building to 3 sets of 5 reps, then 2 sets of 10 and finally 3 sets of 10 reps.

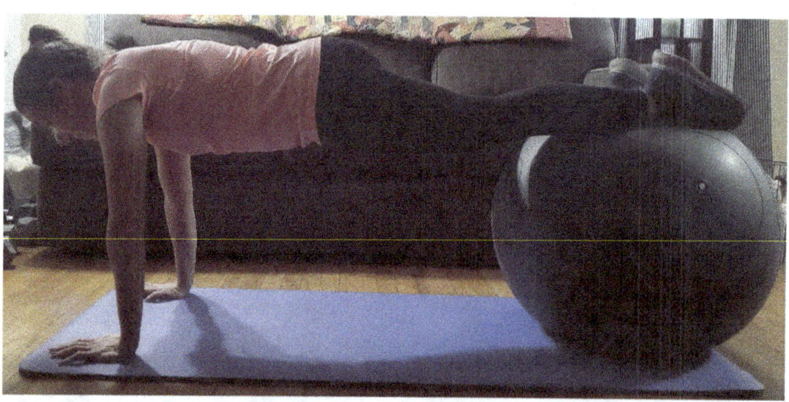

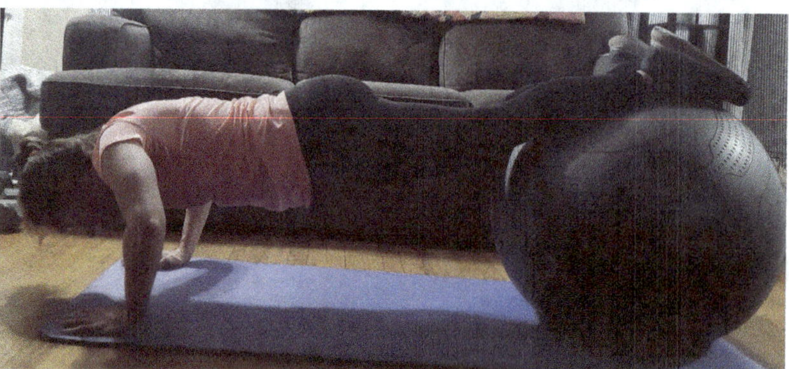

<u>66. Incline Push-Ups</u>
Intermediate

For this exercise, you will be in a plank position with hands on the stability ball and the body out straight with tailbone tucked and toes anchored to the floor. To perform this exercise, you will bend the arms and lower the chest down until it is level with the elbows. Push back up to plank. This completes one rep.

What it Works: This exercise requires that the core stay engaged throughout and the entire upper body will be working to help maintain balance. The primary focus will be on the upper body, especially the muscles of the chest and shoulders.

Begin with 1 set of 5 reps, building to 3 sets of 5 reps, then 2 sets of 10 and finally 3 sets of 10 reps.

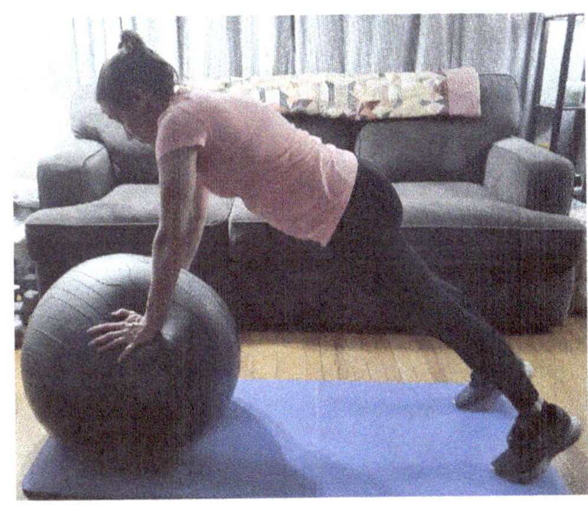

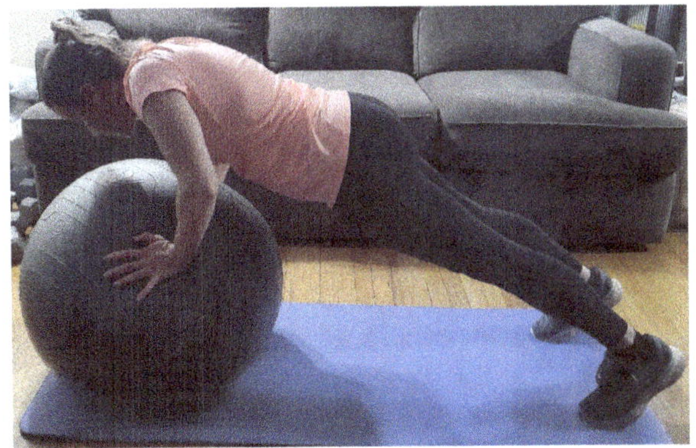

<u>67. One Legged Push-Ups</u>
Intermediate-Advanced

Begin this exercise in a full plank position with hands on the floor and directly under the shoulders, body flat, tailbone tucked and balls of the feet on the stability ball. You will raise one leg up off the stability ball, then perform a push-up by lowering the chest down to elbow height and pushing back up to the start position. The elevated leg will stay elevated throughout the exercise. Repeat evenly on each side.

What it Works: This is a total body exercise that primarily targets the muscles of the upper body including the chest, back and shoulders.

Begin with 1 set of 5 reps, building to 3 sets of 10 reps.

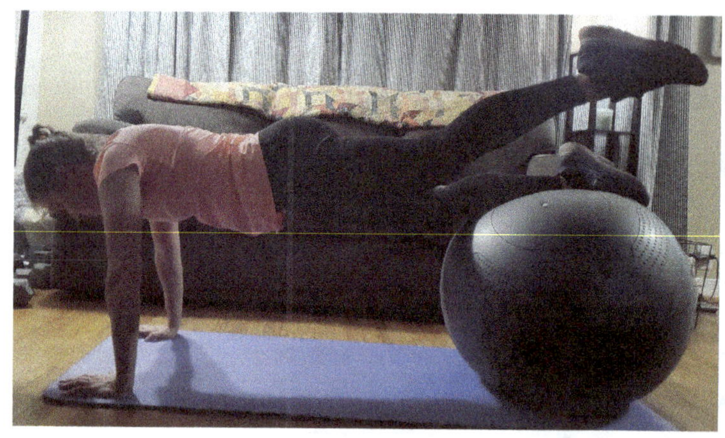

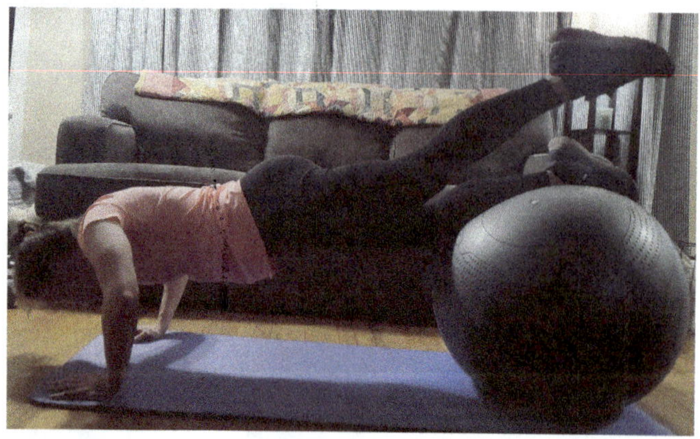

<u>68. Single Arm Sphinx Push-Ups</u>
Intermediate-Advanced

Begin this exercise in the kneeling plank position with knees anchored to the floor and body in a straight line from head to knees with tailbone tucked. Bend one elbow and rest that hand and forearm on the stability ball. Extend the other hand out straight in front of the shoulder and on the floor. To perform this exercise, you will lower the floor side forearm all the way down so that the forearm lies flat on the floor. Push back up to start position. This completes one rep.

What it Works: This exercise really targets the muscles of the upper body, primarily the chest, back and shoulders.

Begin with 1 set of 5 reps, building to 3 sets of 5 reps, then 2 sets of 10 and finally 3 sets of 10 reps.

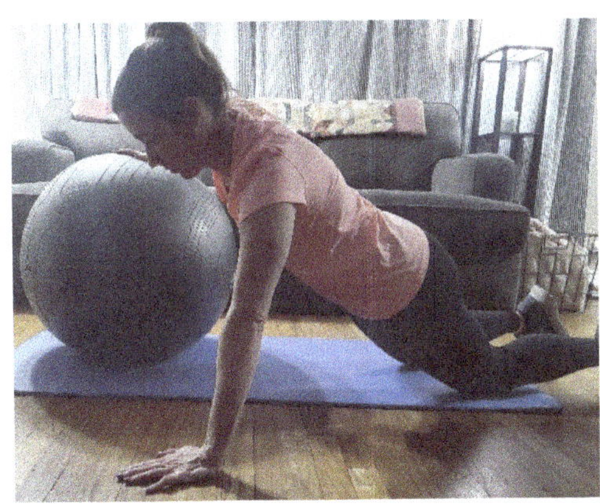

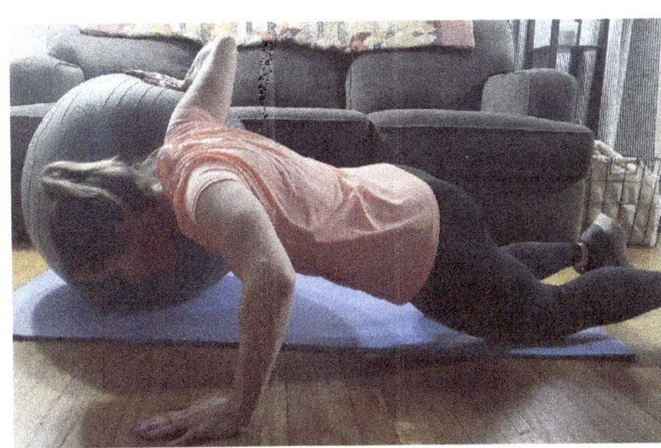

<u>69. Diamond Push-Ups</u>
Intermediate-Advanced

For this exercise you will have the tops of your feet on the stability ball and the hands on the floor. The body will maintain a straight line throughout. The hands will be positioned so that the thumbs and index fingers are touching in a way that creates a diamond shape. You will lower your body down to a push-up by letting the elbows go out to the sides and maintaining the diamond position. Push back up to the start position. This completes one rep.

What it Works: This exercise targets the muscles of the upper body, particularly the chest and arms.

Begin with 1 set of 5 reps, building to 3 sets of 10 reps.

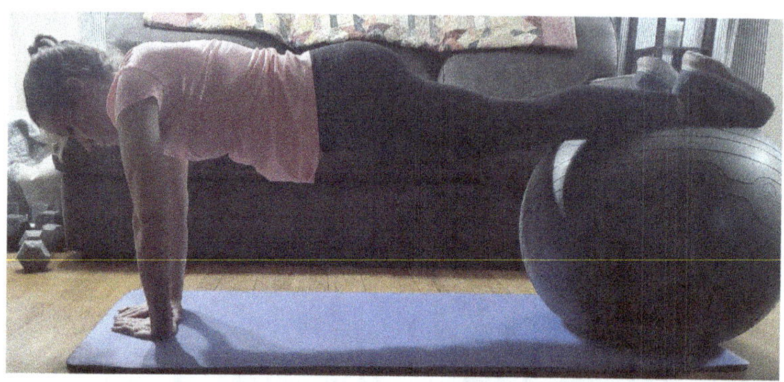

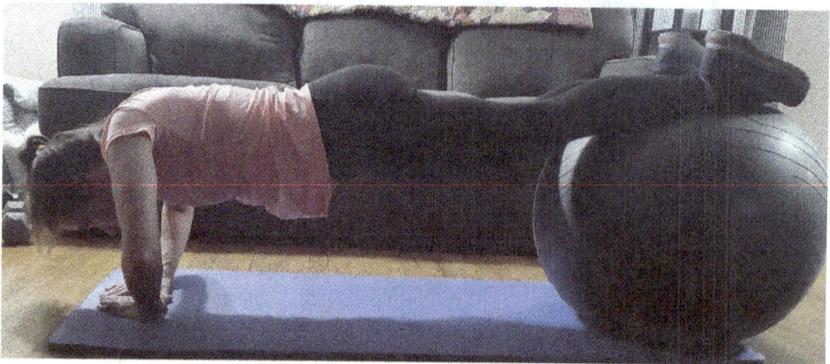

<u>70. Burpees</u>
Intermediate

Your hands will be on the stability ball throughout this multistep exercise. For the first part, you will perform a push up from a full plank position with arms fully extended and body straight. After the push up, you will jump the legs in then reach the stability overhead with outstretched arms as you simultaneously jump up in the air. You will land and simultaneously jump the legs back as the stability ball returns to the floor and you are back in a full plank. This completes one rep.

What it Works: Because of the complexity of this exercise, it engages the total body.

Begin with 1 set of 5 reps, building to 3 sets of 15 reps.

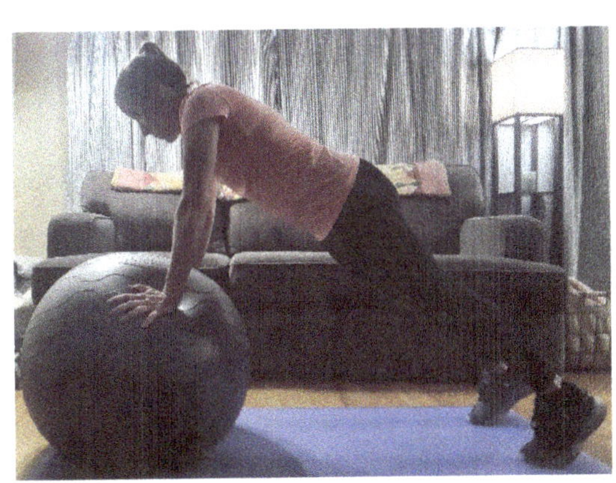

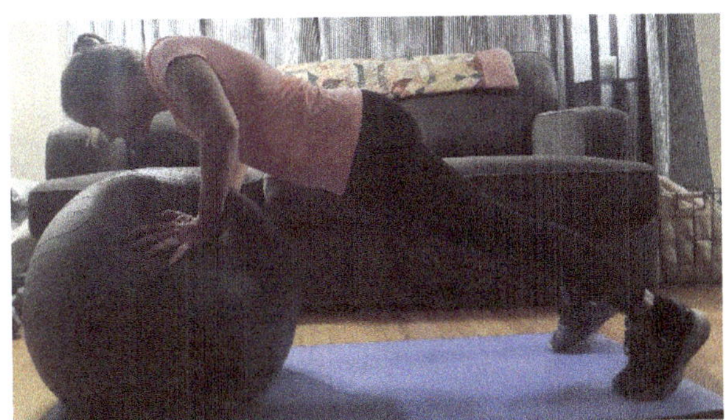

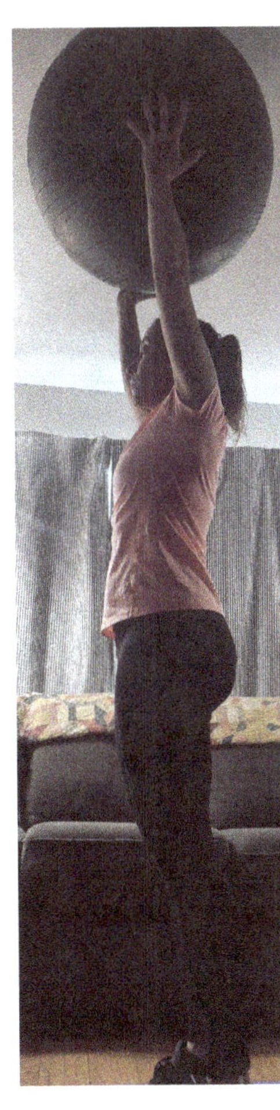

<u>71. Calf Raises</u>
Beginner

Position the stability ball between the chest and the wall with the arms hanging down at your sides. Walk the feet back a bit so that you are leaning into the stability ball while the body maintains a straight line. To perform this exercise, you will raise the heels up off the floor by squeezing the calf muscles and pausing for two counts at the top. Allow the ball to roll down the chest, although this is not a very big movement. Lower back down to the start position. This completes one rep.

What it Works: This exercise targets the calf muscles on the lower backside of the leg.

Begin with 1 set of 10 reps, building to 3 sets of 15 reps.

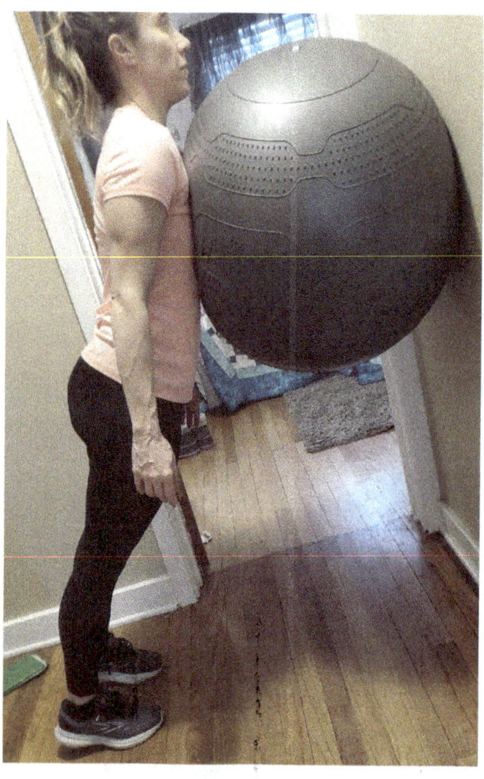 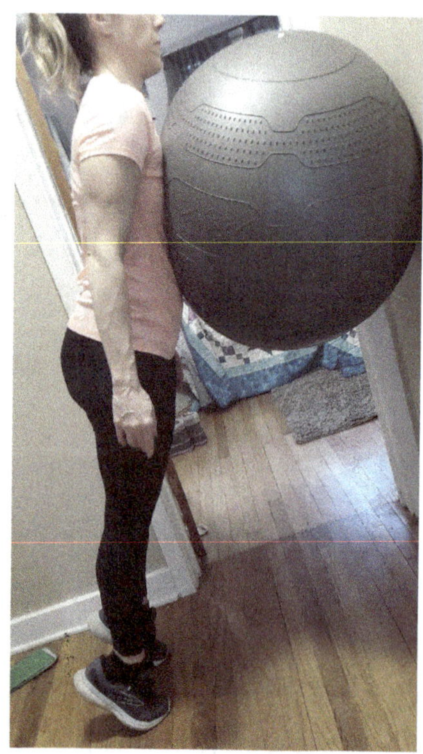

<u>72. Inner Thigh Squeeze</u>
Beginner

Lie flat on your back with knees bent and feet flat on the floor. Position the stability ball between both knees. To perform this exercise, squeeze the stability ball by pressing the knees in. Hold the contraction for 3-5 seconds before releasing. This is one rep.

What it Works: This exercise targets the inner thigh or adductor muscles.

Begin with 1 set of 10 reps, building to 3 sets of 15 reps.

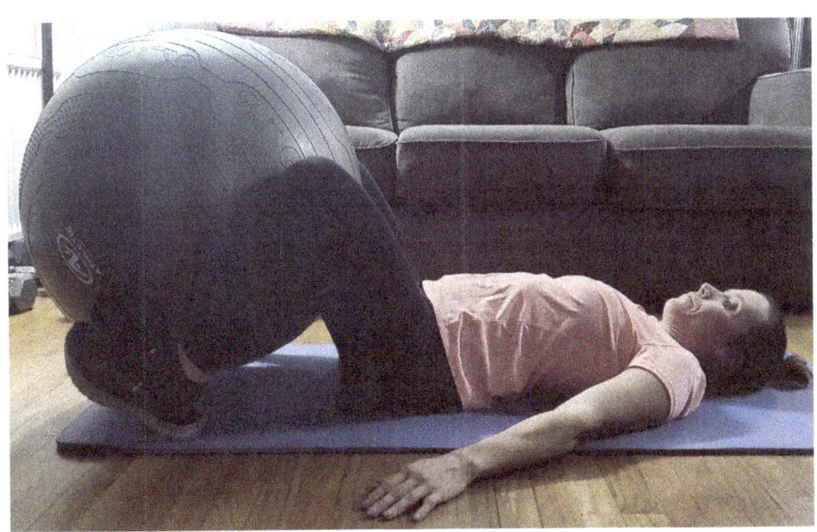

<u>73. Side Leg Lift</u>
Intermediate

Lie on your side and rest your head on your bottom arm. Use your top arm to help stabilize your body by pressing the palm into the floor. The stability ball will be positioned between your ankles and your legs will be stacked and extended out straight. To perform this exercise, you will lift the ball straight up while keeping your legs straight, careful not to allow your hips to roll forward or backward. Hold the ball at the top for 3 seconds before lowering back down. This completes one rep. Repeat evenly on each side.

What it Works: Primarily targets the inner thigh, or adductor muscles.

Begin with 1 set of 5 reps, building to 3 sets of up to 15 reps.

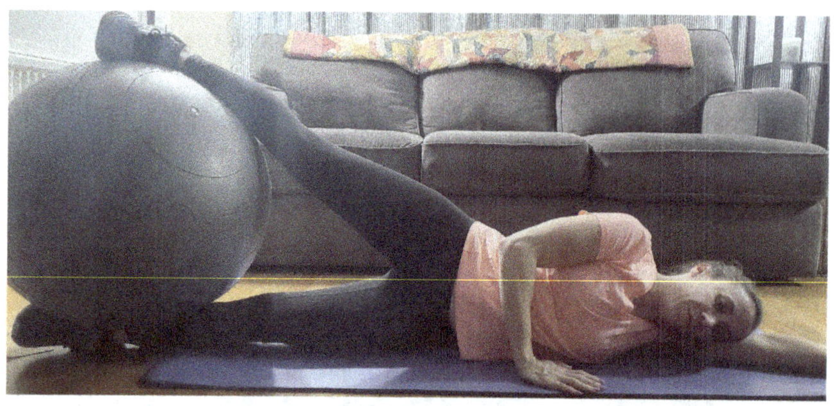

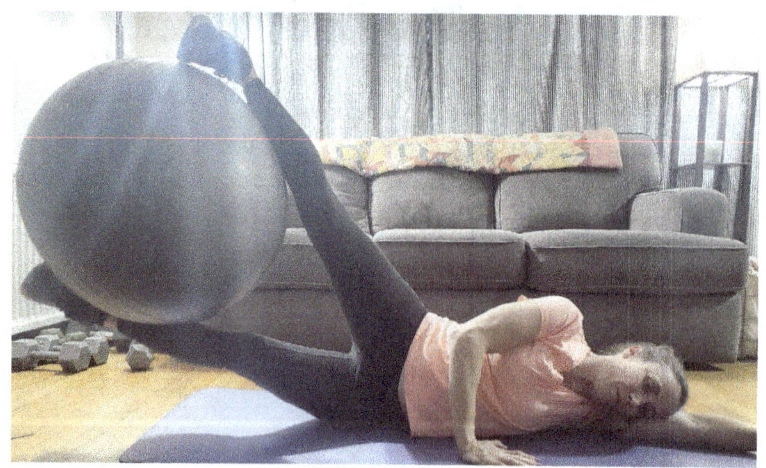

<u>74. Side Plank Leg Lift</u>
Intermediate-Advanced

To begin this exercise, you will be lying with the side of your torso on the stability ball with the bottom arm bent and gripping the ball to help stabilize the body. The feet will be stacked on top of each other and the body will be in a straight line from shoulders to feet. This is the start position. To perform this exercise, you will raise the top leg straight up while being careful not to allow the hips to roll forward or back. The bottom leg and upper body should remain still throughout. Lower back to the start position. This completes one rep. Repeat evenly on each side.

What it Works: This is a total body exercise that engages the core and upper body throughout, but it mainly targets the muscles on the outside of the butt (or glute meds.)

Begin with 1 set of 5 reps, building to 3 sets of 10 reps.

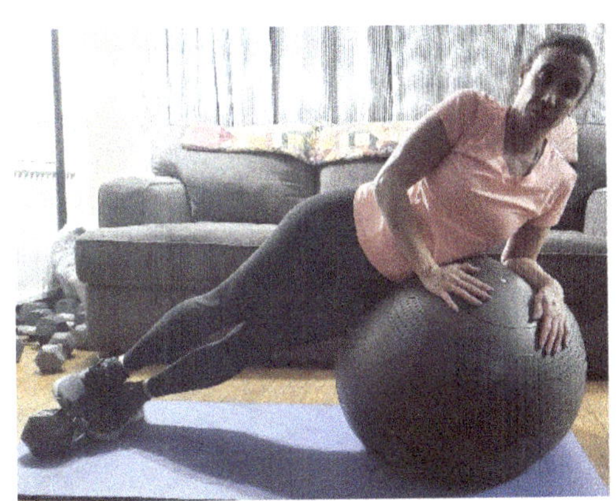

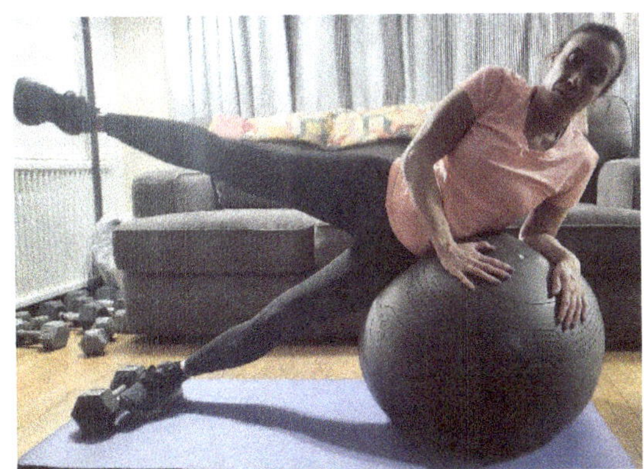

<u>75. Lunge Twist</u>
Beginner

Begin this exercise in a standing position while holding the stability ball in both hands with arms stretched out in front of the chest. You will take a step backwards and lower into a lunge, being careful not to allow the knee of the front leg to go over the toes. As you lunge, you will simultaneously bring the stability ball over to the front leg side by twisting at the waist. The ball will be extended in front of the chest throughout. Come back up to the start position. This completes one rep. Repeat evenly on each side.

What it Works: This is primarily a lower body exercise, although the obliques and shoulders are heavily engaged as well.

Begin with 1 set of 10 reps, building to 3 sets of 10 reps.

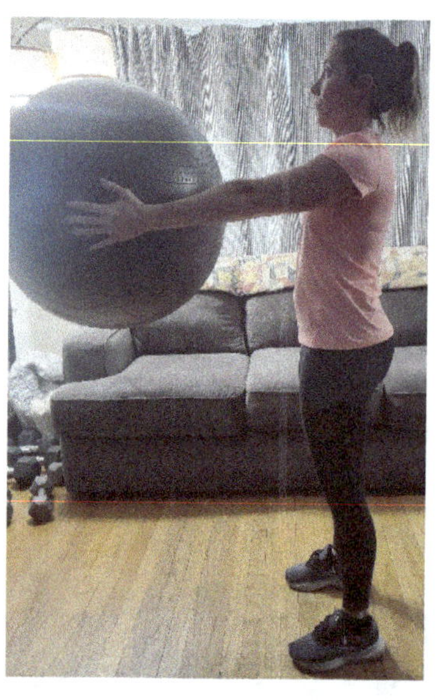
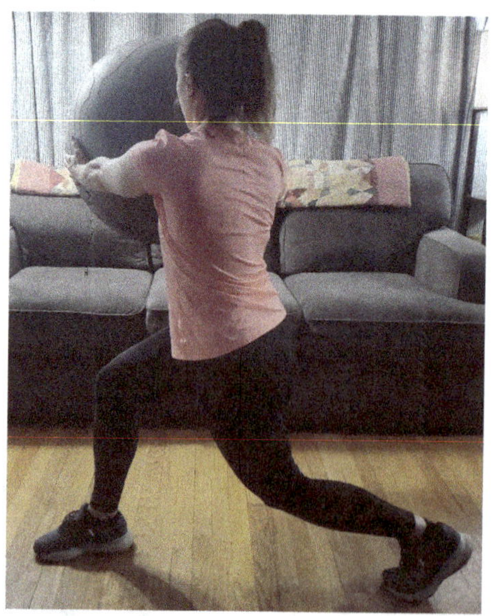

<u>76. Single Leg Deadlift</u>
Beginner

Hold the stability ball in both hands and hold it in outstretched arms in front of the chest. Bend one leg slightly so that all of your weight is on one leg. To perform this exercise, you will lean forward while keeping the standing leg straight and allowing the nonworking leg to drift back. Keep a straight back by hinging at the hips. Hips should stay squared to the front throughout. Come back to standing by pushing through the heel of the anchored leg and contracting the glutes. This completes one rep. Repeat evenly on each leg.

What it Works: This is primarily a lower body exercise that targets the glutes and hamstrings.

Begin with 1 set of 10 reps, building to 3 sets of 10 reps.

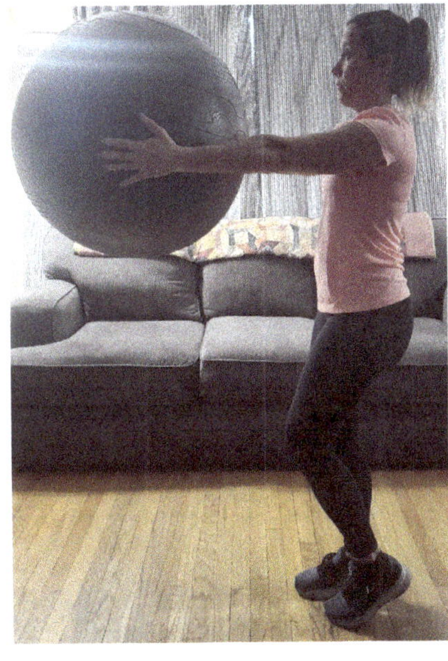 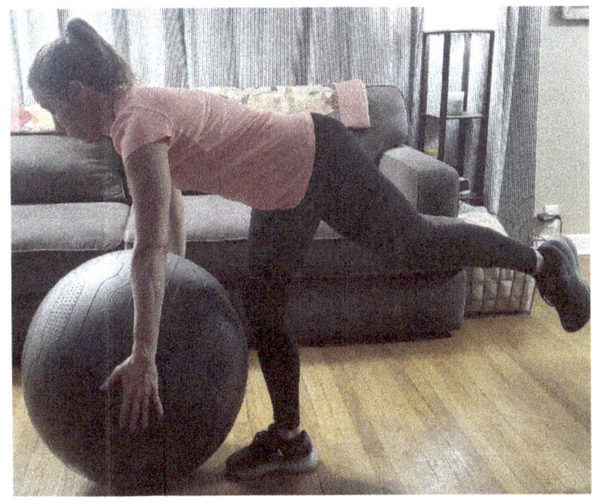

<u>77. Incline Plank Leg Lift</u>
Intermediate

Begin by getting into a hover plank with the forearms and elbows resting on top of the stability ball. The body should be in a straight line from head to heels with the tailbone tucked and the toes anchored to the floor. To perform this exercise, you will lift one leg up so it is hovering above the floor. This leg should not touch the floor again throughout the duration of the set. You will raise the leg straight up, being careful not to arch the back or allow the hips to roll open. Squeeze at the top before lowering back down. This completes one rep. Repeat evenly on each side.

What it Works: Although the core must remain engaged throughout, this is primarily a lower body exercise that really targets the glutes and hamstrings.

Begin with 1 set of 5 reps, building to 3 sets of 10 reps.

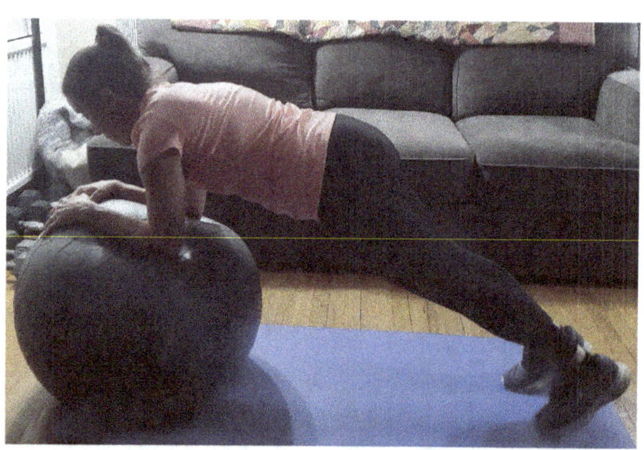

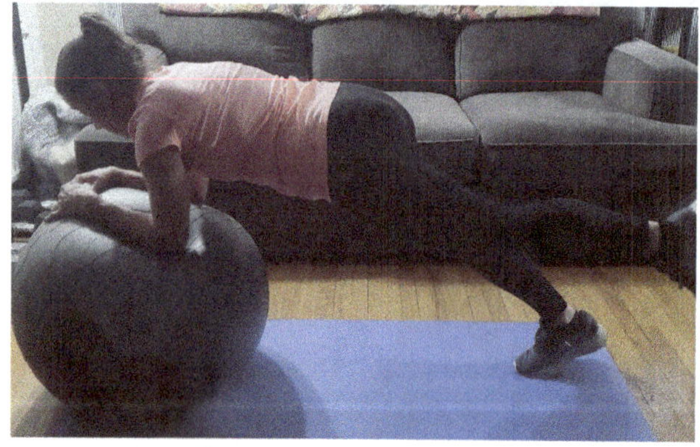

<u>78. Leg Press</u>
Intermediate

From a seated position on the stability ball, walk the feet forward so only the top of the tailbone is on the stability ball. The feet will stay flat on the floor throughout and the arms will hang at your sides. To perform this exercise, you will lower down towards the floor at an incline by bending the knees and allowing the ball to roll up the back. Push back up to the start position at the same incline by driving down through the heels and pushing your back into the stability ball. This completes one rep.

What it Works: This exercise really targets the quads, or the front of the upper leg.

Begin with 1 set of 10 reps, building to 4 sets of 10 reps.

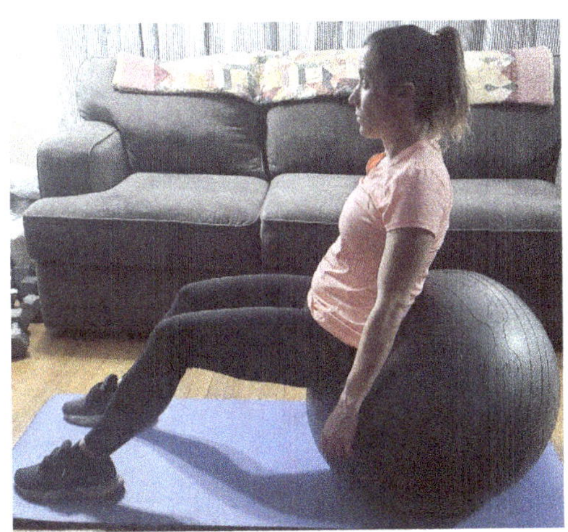

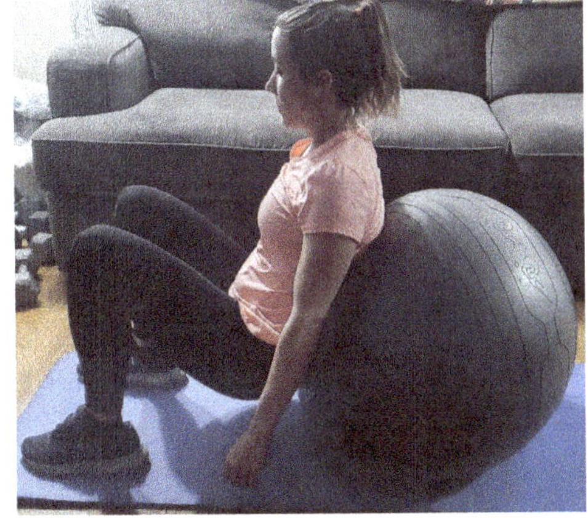

<u>79. Hip Raise</u>
Beginner-Intermediate

Lie flat on your back with your arms down by your sides and your heels on the stability ball. The legs should stay straight throughout. To perform this exercise, you will press down on the palms and the heels while contracting the glutes as you lift your hips up off the floor, stopping when the body is a straight line from feet to shoulders. Lower back down to the start position. This is one rep.

What it Works: This is a lower body exercise that primarily concentrates on the glutes.

Begin with 1 set of 10 reps, building to 3 sets of 10 reps.

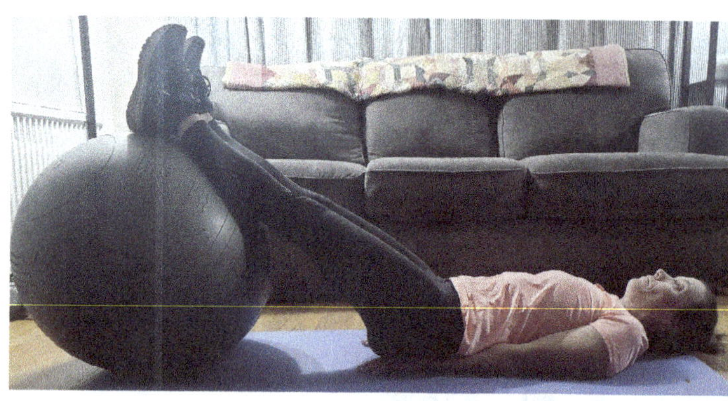

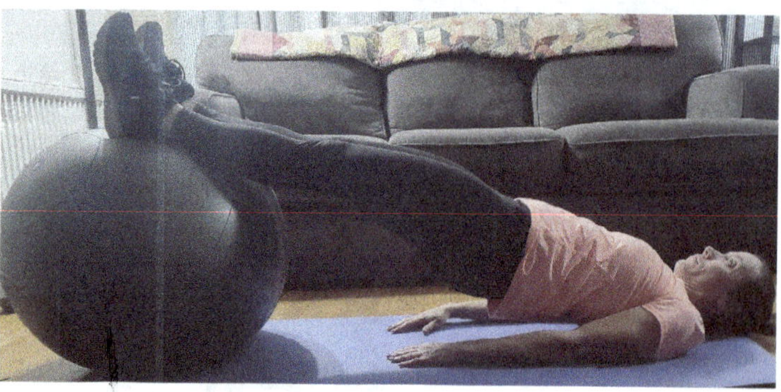

<u>80. One Legged Hip Raise</u>
Intermediate

Lie flat on your back with your arms down by your sides and your heels on the stability ball. The legs should stay straight throughout. Raise one leg above the stability ball. This is the start position. To perform this exercise, you will press down on the palms and the bottom heel while you contract the glute to lift your hips up off the floor, stopping when the bottom leg is in a straight line with the body. Lower down to the start position. This is one rep. Repeat evenly on each side.

What it Works: This is a lower body exercise that primarily concentrates on the glutes.

Begin with 1 set of 5 reps, building to 3 sets of 10 reps.

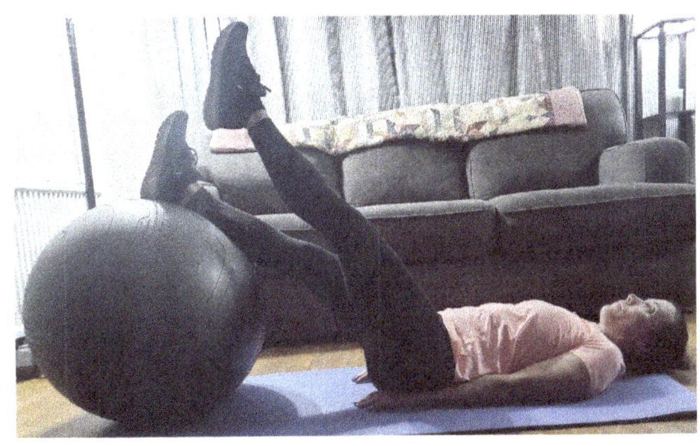

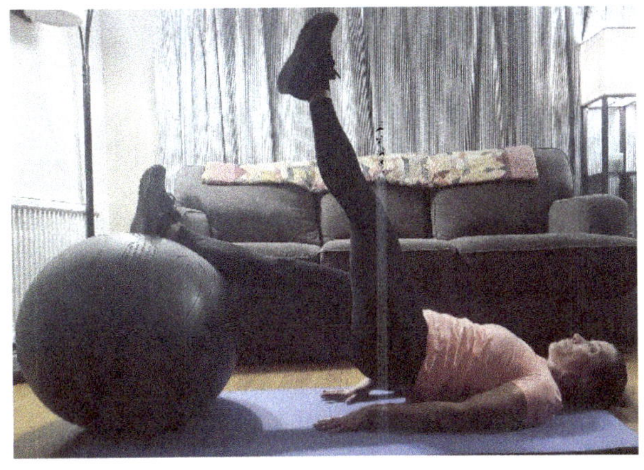

<u>81. Hip Raise Leg Extension</u>
Intermediate

Lie flat on your back and rest your ankles on the stability ball. With arms against the body, raise the hips off the floor while pushing down on the palms, stopping when the body makes a straight line from shoulders to feet. This is the starting position. To perform this exercise, you will bend the knees while pulling the ball in. Stop when the knees are bent at 90 degrees and the feet are flat against the stability ball. Roll back down to the start position. This is one rep.

What it Works: This is a lower body exercise that concentrates on the glutes and hamstrings.

Begin with 1 set of 5 reps, building to 3 sets of 10 reps.

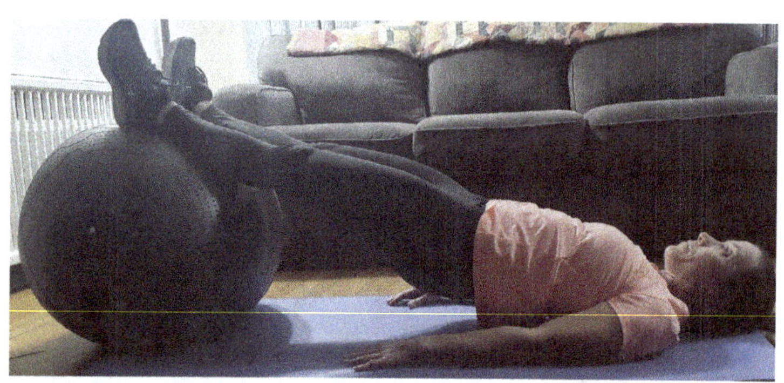

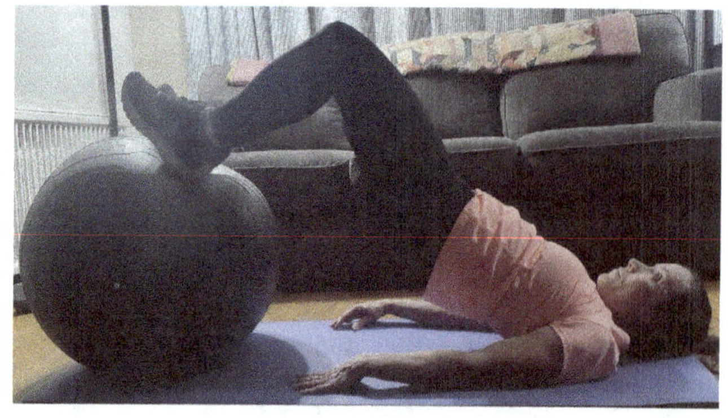

<u>82. Hamstring Squeeze</u>
Intermediate

Begin by lying face down, resting forehead on the forearms and legs outstretched with the stability ball positioned between the ankles/lower legs. The upper body should remain still and anchored to the floor throughout. To perform this exercise, you will raise the legs up straight while squeezing the stability ball between the ankles and engaging the hamstrings. Hold the squeeze at the top for 3 seconds before lowering back down. This completes one rep.

What it Works: This exercise targets the muscles on the backs of the upper legs, or the hamstrings.

Begin with 1 set of 10 reps, building to 3 sets of 10 reps.

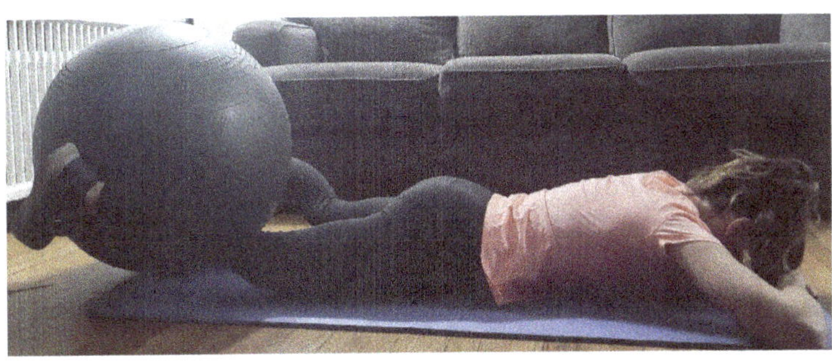

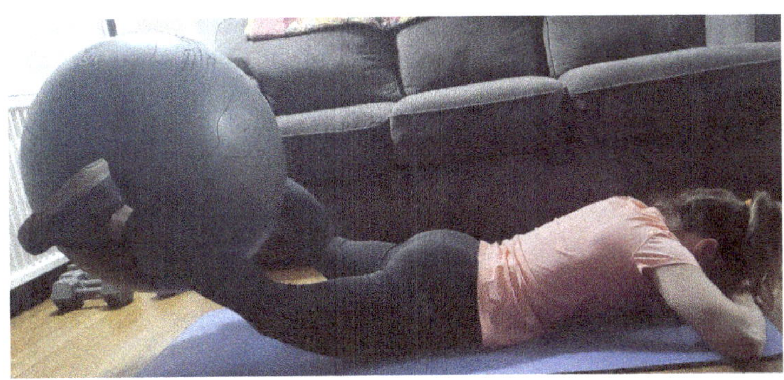

<u>83. Hamstring Tap Outs</u>
Intermediate

Lie flat on your back with arms at your sides, legs stretched out straight with heels on top of the stability ball. Keeping your legs straight, you will raise your hips up off the floor creating a straight line from shoulders to heels. This is the starting position. To perform this exercise, you will first lower one heel over to the side to tap the floor then return to the start position. Repeat on the other side. This completes one rep.

What it Works: The core must remain engaged throughout, but this exercise primarily targets the glutes, hamstrings and hip flexors.

Begin with 1 set of 5 reps, building to 3 sets of 10 reps.

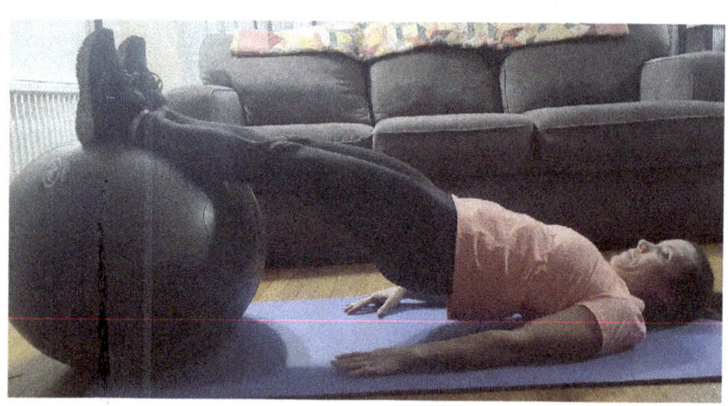

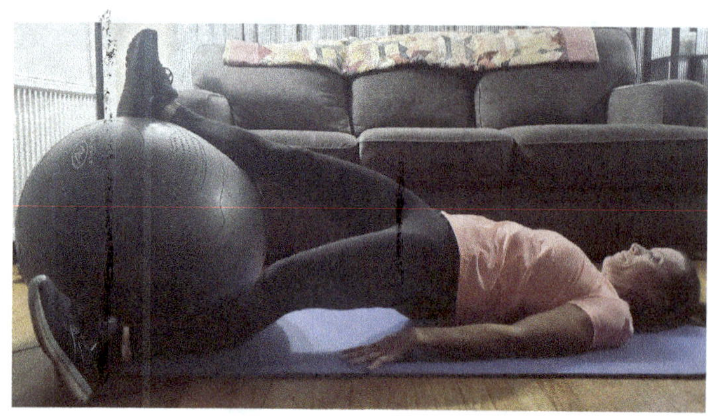

<u>84. V Leg Lifts</u>
Intermediate

Lie face down so the hips are on the stability ball and the hands are on the floor. The legs are extended out straight behind in a V position with feet hovering above the ground. The feet should not touch the floor throughout this exercise. Maintaining the V position with the legs, squeeze the glutes to raise the legs straight up. Lower back to the start position. This completes one rep.

What it Works: This exercise concentrates on the muscles on the back of the leg, particularly the glutes.

Begin with 1 set of 10 reps, building to 3 sets of 10 reps.

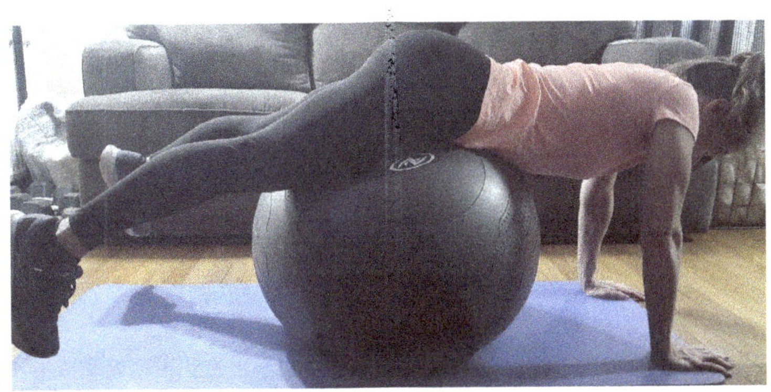

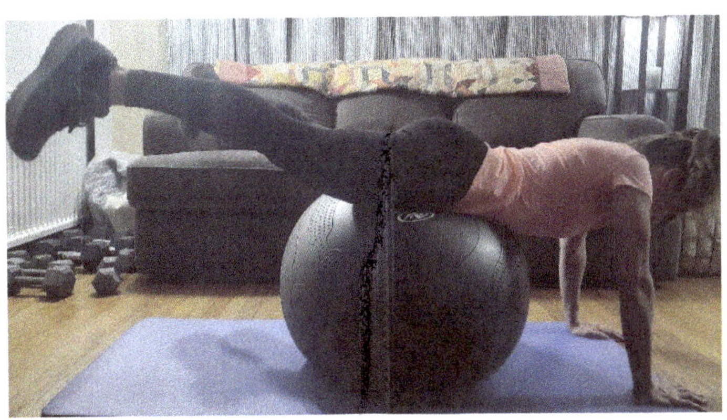

<u>85. Frog Leg Lifts</u>
Intermediate

Lie face down so the hips are on the stability ball and the hands are on the floor. The legs are extended out behind with the knees bent and pointed out to the side with the heels together. While keeping your knees bent in the frog position throughout, you will squeeze the glutes to raise the heels up. Lower back to the start position. This completes one rep.

What it Works: This exercise concentrates on the muscles of the leg, particularly the glutes.

Begin with 1 set of 10 reps, building to 3 sets of 10 reps.

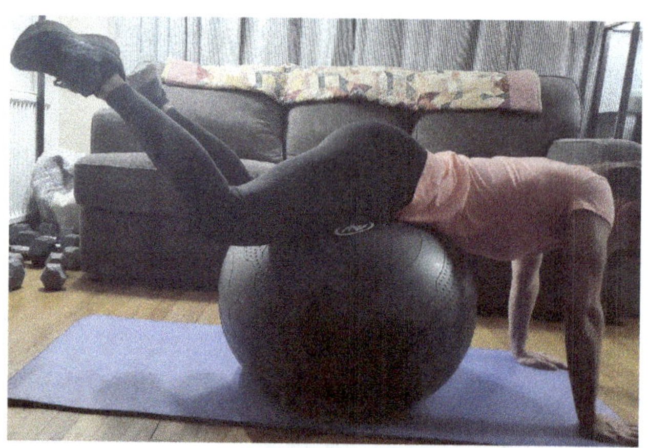

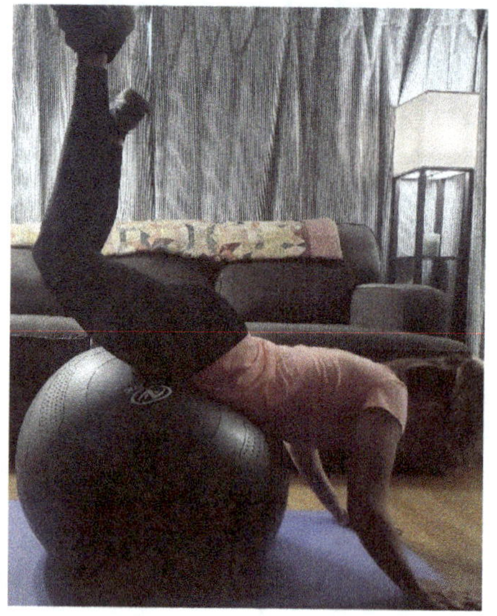

<u>86. Plank Leg Lifts</u>
Intermediate-Advanced

Begin in a forearm plank with the forearms on the stability ball, elbows directly under the shoulders, body in a straight line from head to heels, tailbone tucked and thee balls of the feet anchored to the floor with feet hip width apart. This is the start position. To perform this exercise you will lift one leg straight up, being careful not to let the hips roll to the side or the back arch. Lower back to the start position and repeat on the other leg. This completes one rep.

What it Works: Planks are a total body exercise, but this exercise really targets the glutes.

Begin with 1 set of 5 reps, building to 3 sets of 15 reps.

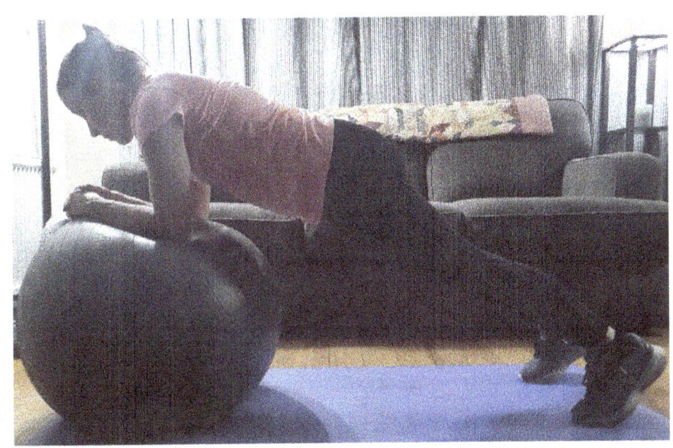

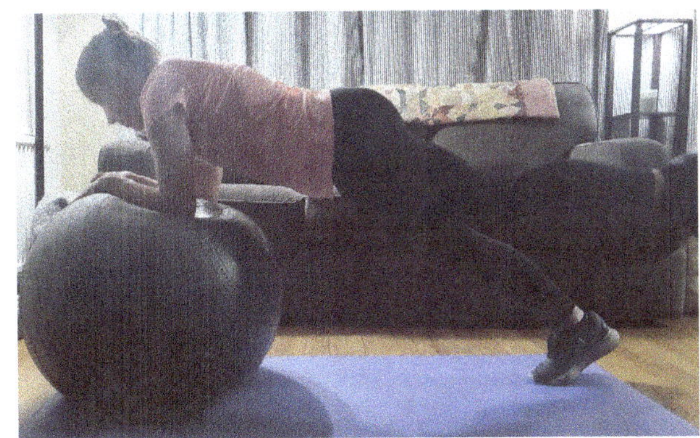

87. Lateral Crab Walks
Beginner-Intermediate

From a seated position on the stability ball, walk the feet forward until the head and shoulders are resting on the ball, the knees are bent at 90 degrees and the torso is flat. To perform this exercise you will walk the feet to one side while allowing the ball to roll over to the same side shoulder. Shuffle the feet back to center then over to the other side before returning to the start position. This completes one rep.

What it Works: This exercise targets the muscles of the glutes and the lower back.

Begin with 1 set of 10 reps, building to 3 sets of 10 reps.

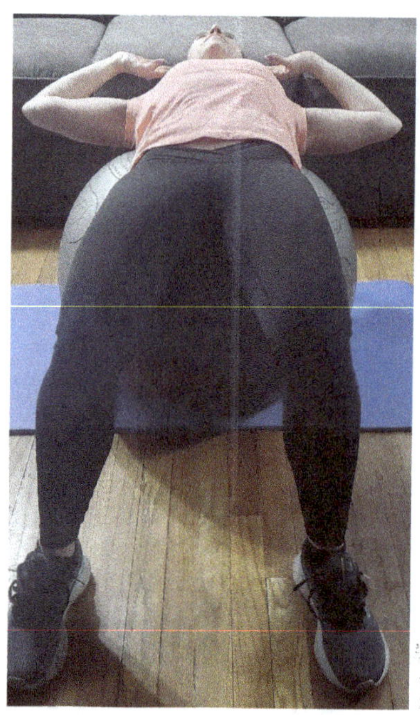 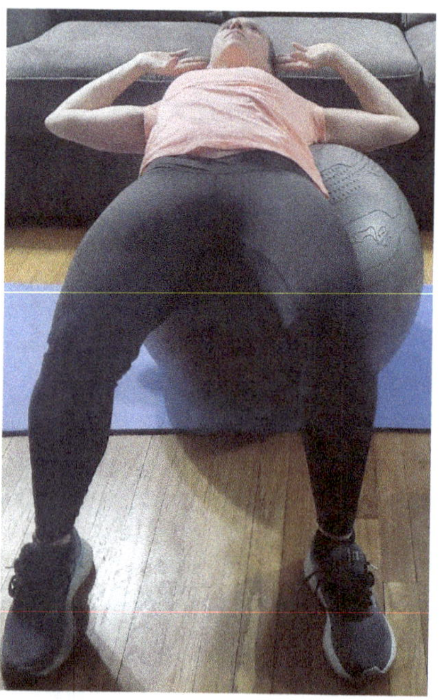

<u>88. Wall Sits</u>
Beginner

Begin this exercise in the set position with your feet hip width apart and the stability ball between the middle of your back and the wall. Your feet should be slightly in front of your body. You will lower down into a squat by rolling your back down the stability ball until your thighs are parallel to the floor. Do not allow the knees to go in front of the toes. This is a static exercise, so you will hold this exercise for a specified amount of time before standing back up.

What it Works: This is a lower body exercise that works the glutes, hamstrings and quads.

Begin by holding for 20 seconds for 1 rep, building to 60 seconds for 3 reps.

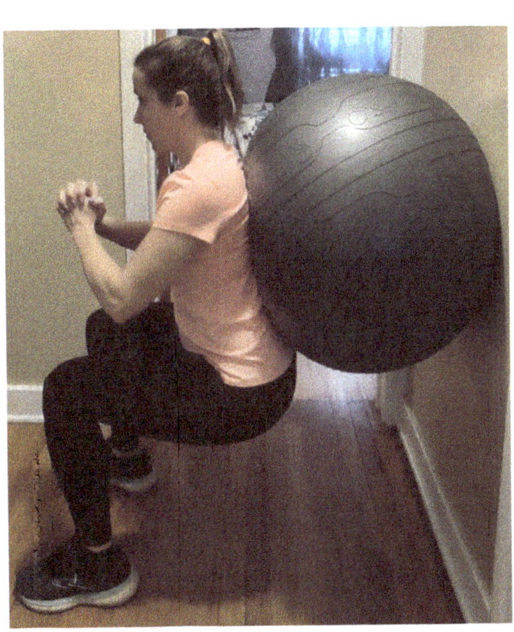

<u>89. Wall Squats</u>
Beginner

Begin this exercise in the set position with your feet hip width apart and the stability ball between the middle of your back and the wall. Your feet should be slightly in front of your body. You will lower down into a squat by rolling your back down the stability ball until your thighs are parallel to the floor. Do not allow the knees to go in front of the toes. Push yourself back up to the start position by driving down through the heels. This is one rep.

What it Works: This is a lower body exercise that works the glutes, hamstrings and quads.

Begin with 1 set of 10 reps, building to 3 sets of 10 reps.

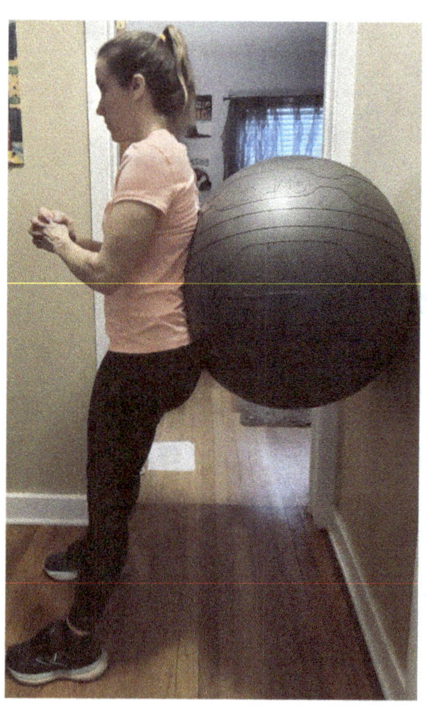 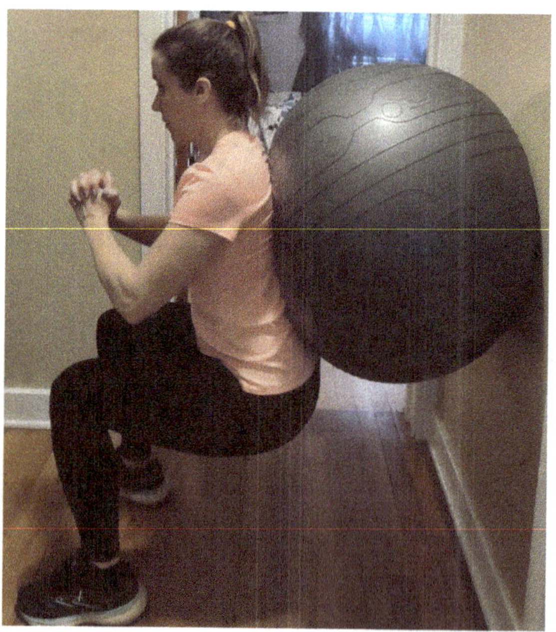

<u>90. Sumo Wall Squats</u>
Beginner

Begin this exercise in a standing position with the feet in an extra wide stance. The feet should be wider than the shoulders and the toes should be pointed out diagonally and in front of the body. The stability ball will be between the middle of your back and the wall. You will lower down into a squat by rolling the stability ball up your back, making sure the knees follow the line of the toes, but not bending so as to go beyond them. Push yourself back to the start position by driving through the heels. This is one rep.

What it Works: This is a lower body exercise that targets the glute meds, or the outer gluteal muscle.

Begin with 1 set of 10 reps, building to 3 sets of 10 reps.

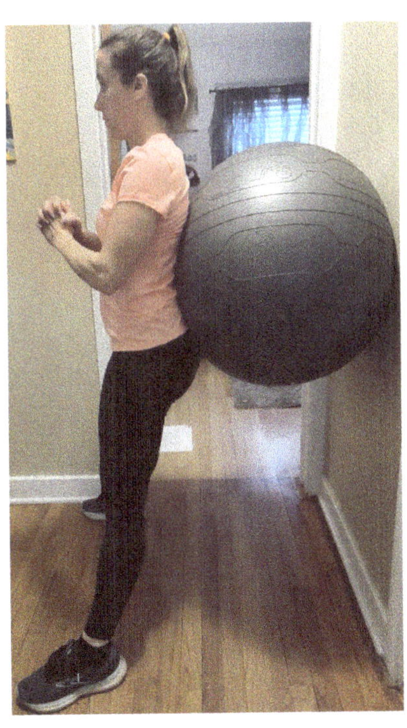 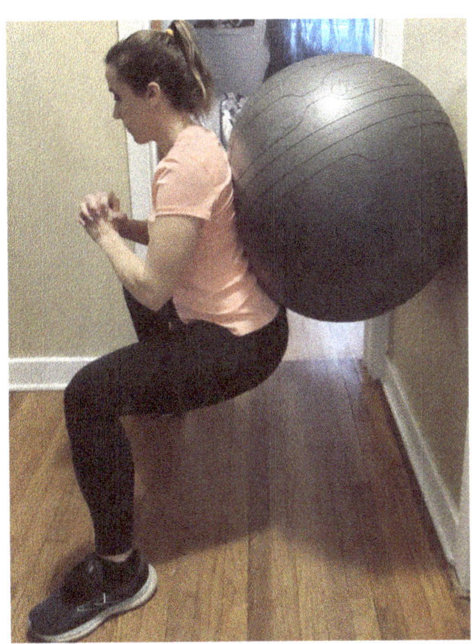

<u>91. Single Leg Wall Squats</u>
Intermediate-Advanced

Begin this exercise in the set position with your feet hip width apart and the stability ball between the middle of your back and the wall. Your feet should be slightly in front of your body. Raise one leg so that it is extended out straight in front of you. This is the starting position. Next, you will lower down into a squat by driving down through the standing heel and while allowing the ball to roll up the back. Push back up to the starting position. This completes one rep. Repeat evenly on each side.

What it Works: This is a lower body exercise that concentrates on the glutes, hamstrings and quads.

Begin with 1 set of 5 reps, building to 3 sets of 10 reps.

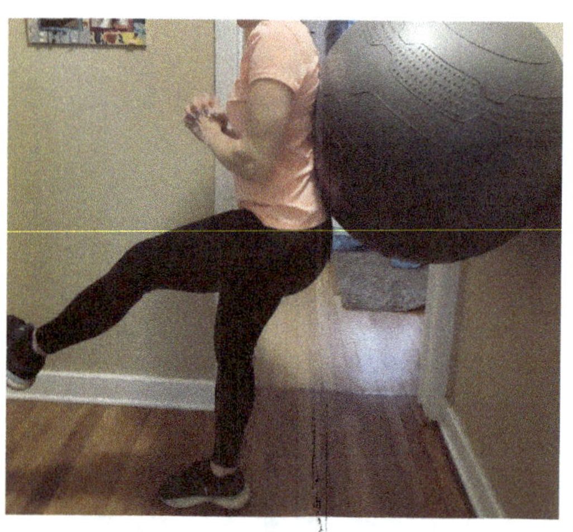
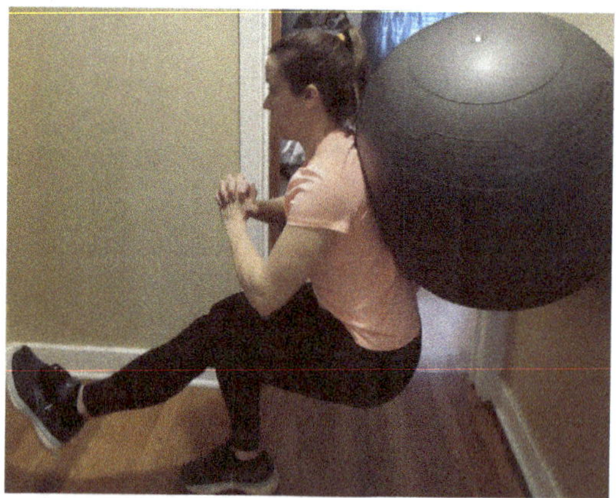

<u>92. Atlas Squats</u>
Beginner

From a standing position with feet shoulder width apart and toes pointed out diagonally, you will hold the stability ball in both hands and raise it straight up overhead. Lower down into a deep squat by driving the hips back and down, being careful not to allow the knees to cover the toes. The stability ball stays overhead throughout. Push back up to the start position by driving down through the heels. This completes one rep.

What it Works: This is primarily a lower body exercise, although the upper body is also engaged throughout.

Begin with 1 set of 10 reps, building up to 3 sets of 15 reps.

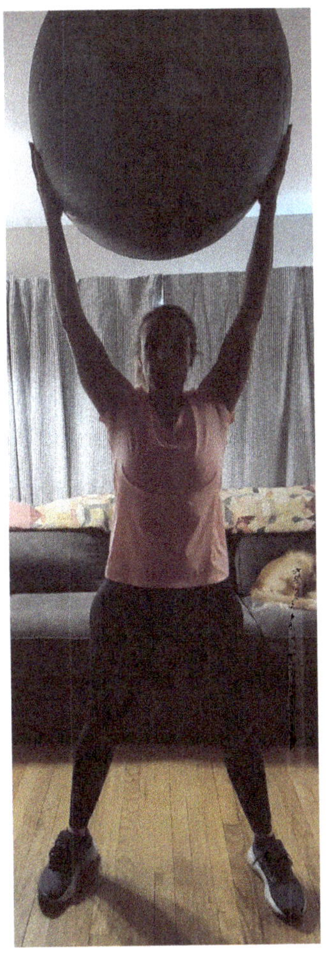 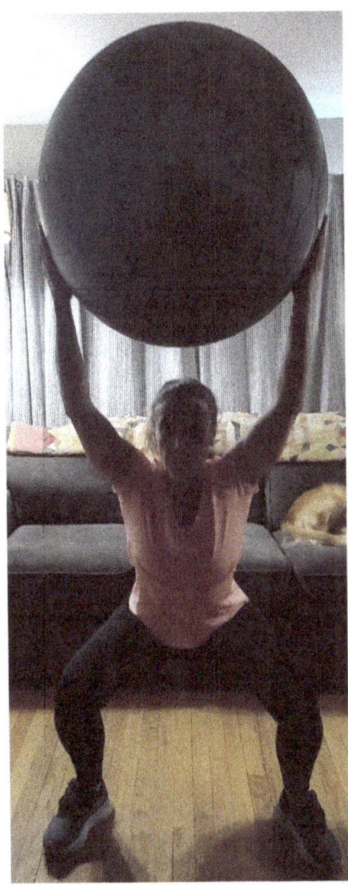

<u>93. Reverse Bridge</u>
Beginner-Intermediate

Lie flat on back and bend knees at a 90 degree angle, resting the bottoms of the feet on the stability ball. By pushing the back down into the floor and the feet into the stability ball, lift the hips up off the floor until the body forms a straight line from shoulders to knees. Lower back down. This completes one rep.

What it Works: This exercise engages the core, but is predominantly targeting the glutes.

Begin with 1 set of 5 reps, building to 3 sets of 5 reps, then 2 sets of 10 and finally 3 sets of 10 reps.

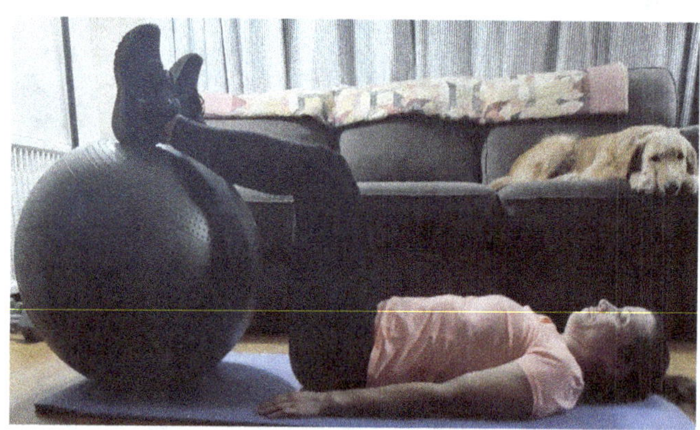

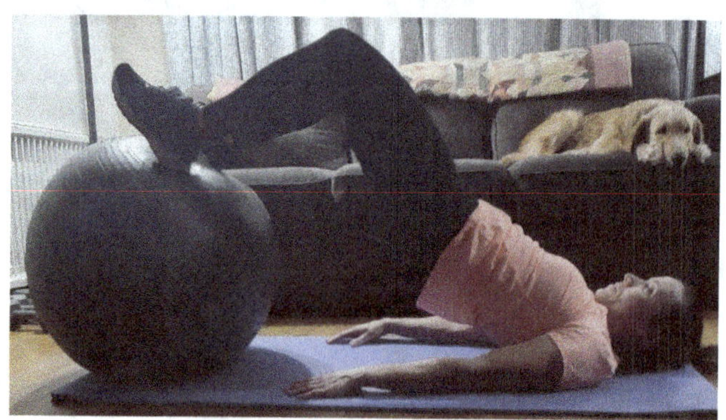

<u>94. Hip Thrusts</u>
Beginner-Intermediate

Begin this exercise by pressing the upper back against the stability ball, knees bent and feet flat on the floor. Arms will be bent out to the sides with hands at the temples and hips will be hovering above the floor. To perform this exercise, you will press your back into the stability ball, drive down through the heels and lift the hips up by squeezing the glutes until the thighs are parallel with the floor. Lower back down to start. This is one rep.

What it Works: This exercise concentrates on the gluteal muscles.

Begin with 1 set of 5 reps, building to 3 sets of 5 reps, then 2 sets of 10 and finally 3 sets of 10 reps.

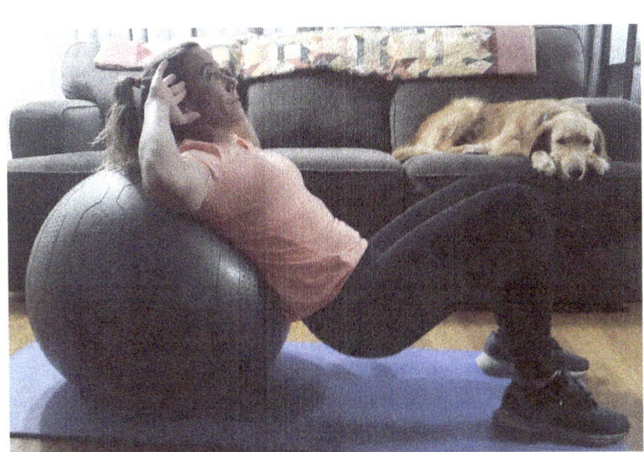

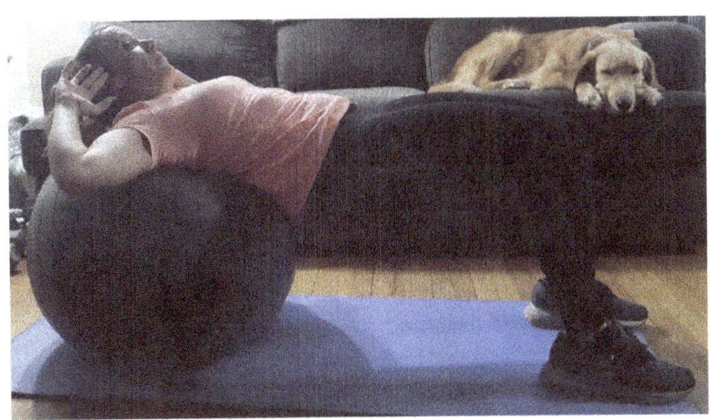

<u>95. Decline Plank Leg Lift</u>
Intermediate

You will maintain a plank position throughout this exercise, with arms stretched out straight, hands flat on the floor directly under the shoulders, and legs stretched out straight with the shins resting on the stability ball. The body should be a straight line with a flat back and tailbone tucked. To perform this exercise, you will lift one leg straight up while maintaining an even plank. Return to the start position and repeat on the other side. This completes one rep.

What it Works: Planks are a total body exercise with an emphasis on the shoulders and core, but the use of the stability ball creates a focus on the gluteal muscles.

Begin with 1 set of 5 reps, building to 3 sets of 5 reps, then 2 sets of 10 and finally 3 sets of 10 reps.

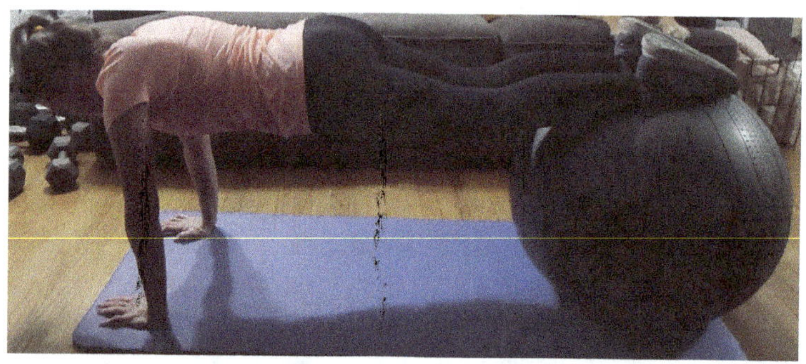

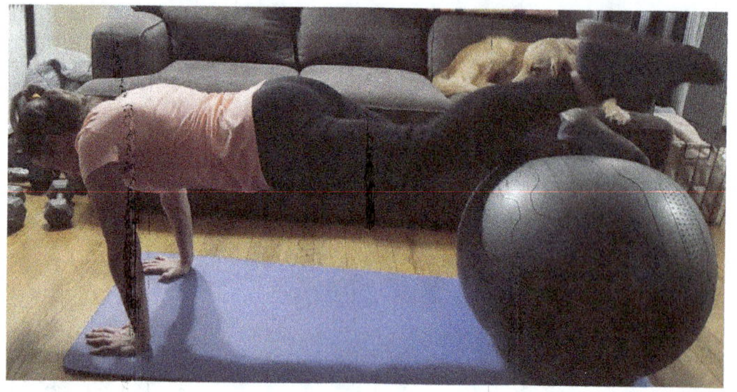

96. Cossack Squats
Intermediate

From a standing position, you will bring the inside of one foot up to rest on top of the stability ball. The other foot will remain anchored to the floor. To perform this exercise, you will allow the stability ball to roll out to the side as the anchored leg lowers into a squat by driving the hip back and down and being careful not to allow the knee to go over the toes. Do not allow the hip on the anchored leg to push out to the side. Push back up to standing by driving through the heel. This completes one rep. Repeat evenly on each side.

What it Works: This is a lower body exercise that targets the hip adductors, quads, glutes and hamstrings.

Begin with reps.

1 set of 5 reps, building up to 3 sets of 10 reps.

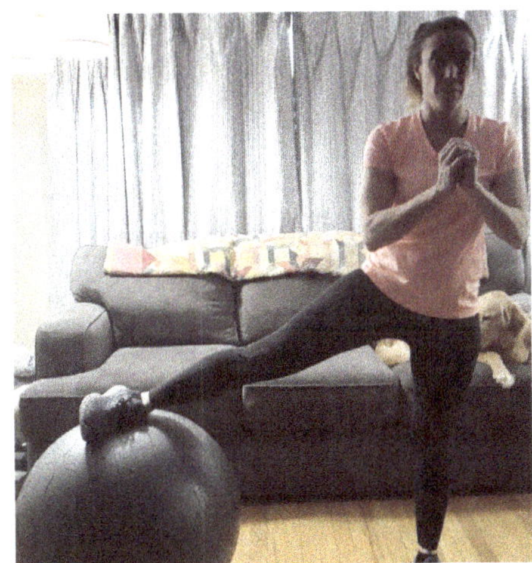

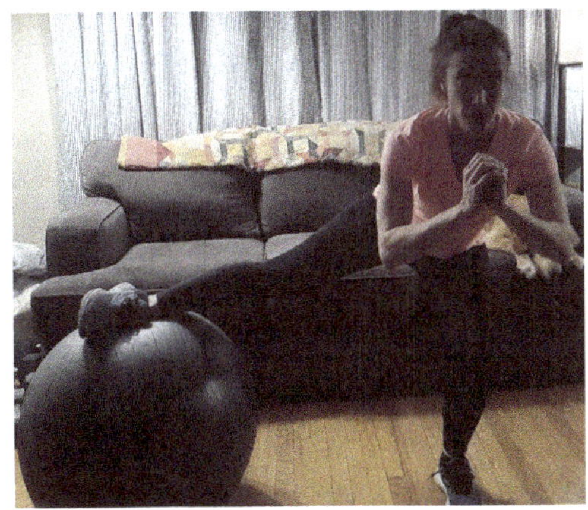

<u>97. Bulgarian Squats</u>
Advanced

To perform this exercise, you are going to begin in a standing set position with one leg extended behind you and resting the top of the foot on the stability ball. Roll the ball far enough back that you are able to squat the front the leg down while keeping the knee behind the toes. You are going to lower straight down, then push back up by driving your weight through the front heel. Try to keep the ball steady. Repeat the exercise evenly on each side.

What it Works: This is primarily a lower body exercise. It is an advanced exercise that requires balance and engages the core throughout. The main muscles that are worked are the posterior muscles of the upper leg (hamstrings and glutes.)

Begin with 1 set of 5 reps, building to 3 sets of 5 reps, then 2 sets of 10 and finally 3 sets of 10 reps.

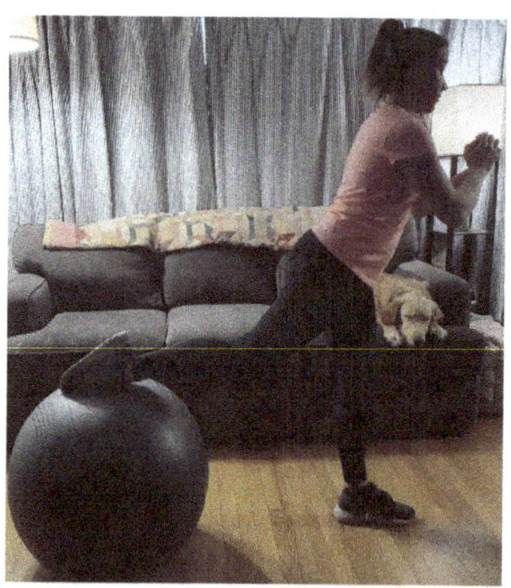

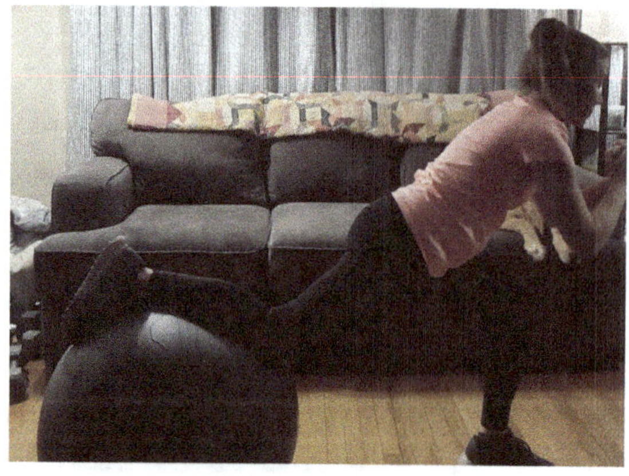

<u>98. Alternating Kicks</u>
Intermediate-Advanced

Lying on your back, you will position the stability ball so it's under both feet. To perform this exercise, you will raise your hips off the floor into a reverse bridge. The hips will stay elevated throughout. Straighten one leg and point it towards the ceiling as you drive the other heel into the stability ball. Bend that leg back down as the heel returns to the stability ball. Repeat on the other side. This completes one rep.

What it Works: This is a lower body exercise that really targets the backs of the legs, or the hamstrings, as well as the glutes.

Begin with 1 set of 5 reps, building to 3 sets of 5 reps, then 2 sets of 10 and finally 3 sets of 10 reps.

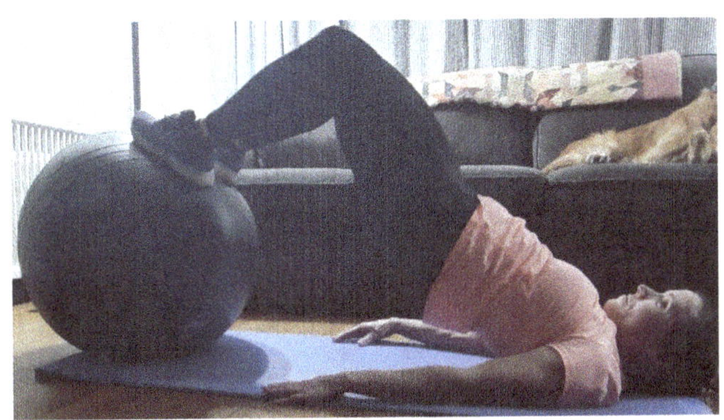

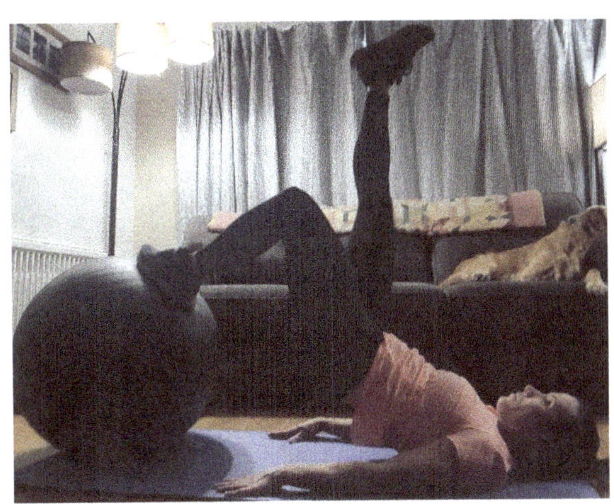

<u>99. Reaching Rear Lunge</u>
Intermediate-Advanced

From a standing position, bring one foot back to rest on top of the stability ball. To perform this exercise, you will hinge forward at the hips bending the anchored leg while the raised leg rolls the stability ball backwards. You want to lower down as low as you can without rolling your back before pushing back up by driving through your anchored heel. This completes one rep. Repeat evenly on each side.

What it Works: This is a lower body exercise that targets the hamstrings and glutes.

Begin with 1 set of 5 reps, building up to 3 sets of 10 reps.

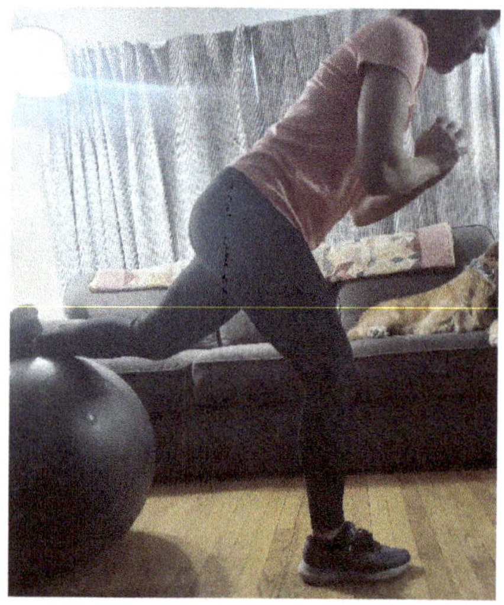
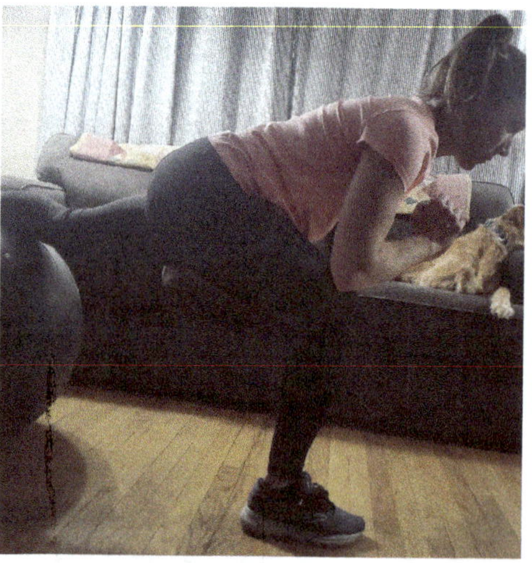

<u>100. Single Leg Hip Thrusts</u>
Intermediate

Lie flat on the floor with knees bent at 90 degrees and heels of feet on the stability ball. Arms will stay at sides throughout helping to stabilize the body. To begin this exercise, extend one leg and raise the foot straight up into the air. This is the starting position. Next you will raise the hips up off the ground while driving the upper back down into the floor and the heel of the foot into the stability ball. Pause at the top when the body has made a straight line from the knee down the torso before lowering back to the start position. This is one rep. Complete evenly on each side.

What it Works: This is an advanced exercise that really targets the glutes and hamstrings.

Begin with 1 set of 5 reps, building to 3 sets of 10 reps.

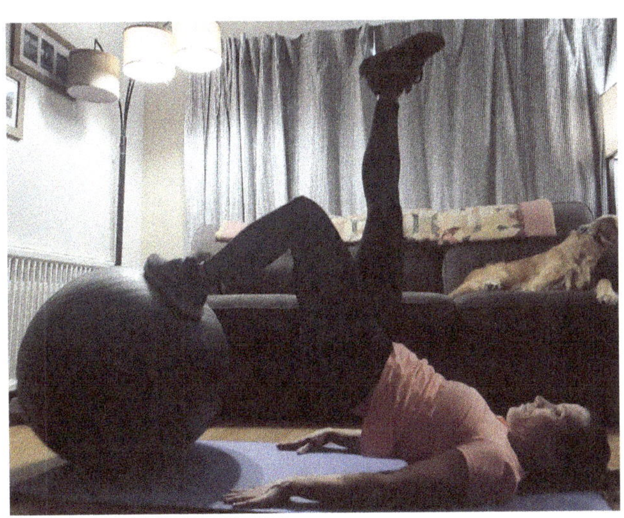

www.ingramcontent.com/pod-product-compliance
Lightning Source LLC
Chambersburg PA
CBHW080853260726
48660CB00009B/3298